Life in Balance

Other Lifeflow® publications

Also by Graham Williams

Insight and Love An introduction to Insight Meditation:
a practical way to become free from emotional conflict

Experience Yourself a CD of guided meditations

Reflections in Water a CD of piano music of Debussy, Chopin and Liszt

My Heart Keeps Watch a CD of piano music of Olivier Messiaen

The Joy of Being a set of four CDs with meditations from the
introductory course and music by renowned Australian composer,
Ross Edwards, in conjunction with ABC Classics.

The Lifeflow Meditation Centre also offers:

- Four terms of courses each year from Level 1 to Level 4
- Retreats and workshops at Tara Hills Retreat Centre
- Customised meditation training courses at our studio or at workplaces
- Corporate programs
- Courses and sessions for schools
- Personal consultations to guide your meditation practice
- Courses for meditation guides
- Teacher training programs

For further information see the end of this book or contact:

The Lifeflow Meditation Centre
Unit 8 / 259 Glen Osmond Rd, Frewville SA 5063, Australia
Ph (61) 08 8379 9001
www.lifeflow.com.au

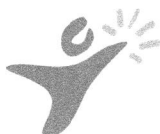

the **Life**flow
meditation centre

life in balance

Life in Balance

The Lifeflow Guide to Meditation

A practical Australian handbook
for understanding and getting
what you want from
your meditation practice

GRAHAM WILLIAMS Ph.D.

Lifeflow® Meditation Centre
Unit 8 / 259 Glen Osmond Rd,
Frewville SA 5063, Australia

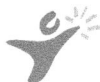

the **Life**flow
meditation centre

ISBN: 978-0-9804562-1-9

Printed in Australia by Print Know How, Unley, South Australia

Cover and book design by Michael Cannon: www.designeye.com.au

Cover image: detail of *Time* by kind permission of the artist Garry Duncan

To my parents Ken and Margaret Williams,
with love and gratitude
for their devotion to each other
and the security this provided.

About the author

Graham Williams was born in Australia. A concert pianist and teacher, he graduated from the University of Adelaide with a Ph.D. and Grad. Dip. Ed. and taught there for 15 years. While studying in Paris he realised that music was one of the few living traditions of meditation in the West. This led him to over ten years' training as a teacher in both the Burmese and Tibetan meditation traditions, and six years in intensive retreat. He has concentrated on bringing the advanced techniques of these incredibly rich traditions into an easily accessible form.

Graham has created a uniquely Australian form of meditation which embraces the rich natural environment and Australian art and music. He is founder and director of the Lifeflow Meditation Centre and has been teaching meditation for over 25 years. He has trained a team of seven teachers who now work together in the Centre, which has taught thousands of people how to meditate and trained hundreds in the more advanced practices.

Graham is also an Adjunct Lecturer in the School of Medicine at Flinders University and a consultant to a national company of corporate psychologists and still teaches piano.

His retreats in the mallee country of South Australia, near the River Murray, have engendered a love of this timeless, peaceful land and he has become a passionate advocate for the conservation of this unique part of Australia's heritage.

This book is the first in a series of four based on the curriculum of the Centre.

Acknowledgments

My editor, Gretta Koch, has provided invaluable support in her tireless and patient quest to prune and tidy up my writing. As both a student and teacher in the Lifeflow Meditation Centre she has a full and clear understanding of meditation and I am deeply indebted to her for her work on this book.

John Burston and Ann Calvert, both long-standing teachers in the Centre whose friendship I value greatly, have been generous in discussing the ideas presented in this book and helping to formulate the curriculum of the Centre. Lisa Hancock, our administrative officer has been, as always, a good friend and an enormous support.

I would also like to thank my brother, Dr David Williams, and Janine Koch for kindly giving their time to read through the text and share their suggestions and ideas.

My friend, the artist Garry Duncan, has given more than he realises in allowing us to use the images of his paintings both on the covers of CDs and books and for our visualisations.

I would like to thank my colleague Eric Harrison for generously sharing his teaching experience. Although we developed the concept of Spot Meditations quite independently, I am indebted to him for the name (I used to call them "quickies").

I've learned a lot from students and clients over the years and am grateful to them for this privilege. I have shared some of their experiences in this book but have maintained anonymity to respect their privacy.

Finally, I would like to express my deep and lasting gratitude to my teachers; in meditation: Namgyal Rinpoche, H.H. the 16th Karmapa and Sharpa Choeje Lobsang Rinpoche; in philosophy: Dene Barnett; in psychotherapy: Dr Earle Williams; and in music: the composers Olivier Messiaen and Richard Meale and the pianists Yvonne Loriod, Germaine Mounier and Lance Dossor.

LIFE IN BALANCE

Contents

Prologue

Discovering meditation

Meditation has been part of my life for a long time now and I still find it an incredibly beautiful and blissful thing to do. I first learned to meditate thirty years ago while training to be a concert pianist in Paris. Living and working in Paris was exciting but also stressful. I enjoyed the intensity of the life, the singleness of purpose, the concentration it was possible to develop and the stimulating relationships with my teachers and fellow students. However, it meant that nearly every hour of every day was taken up with work and I got used to living like this, as do many musicians.

When I joined my class, one of the new students, a Canadian, came over to me and said, "Hi, I've got a teacher and you're going to be interested". I was bemused by this as he looked like a hippy and I had absolutely no interest in what I saw as the hippy, guru world. However, as I got to know him I liked him and we became friends. I respected his knowledge of music and his work as a composer.

He pointed out that I was very tense and this amazed me. I had never viewed myself in this way at all—it was normal. So I decided to learn to meditate as he suggested. We arranged to meet each week at his place where he and his wife taught me meditation and yoga exercises. Along with this went a meal we all contributed to, with the best wine we could afford on our limited student budgets.

While playing piano in my room, trying to get an extremely difficult piece that was driving me crazy ready for the next lesson, I decided to put to the test what I had learned. In the heat of the moment I sat down and watched my breath as I had been taught. I was amazed at what happened. Immediately the tension in my head and shoulders disappeared, my stomach relaxed, and the incredible pressure I was under dissolved.

It was instant! My mind cleared, my emotions settled down and after fifteen minutes I went back to the piano and saw the piece in a completely different light. Instead of battling with it, as I had been doing, I found I could watch it and was able to remain clear and concentrated while working with its complexities.

Music as meditation

As my lessons progressed with my piano teacher, it became clear that she was expecting me to stop thinking about what I was playing and *just play*. Piling on the pressure was one way to make this happen. The moment of illumination came when she suddenly cried out while I was playing, "Stop thinking!" She caught the moment I started to think about what I was doing, and thus lose the plot. In all my years of study, no-one had ever suggested anything like this, but it changed everything.

I could see the effect thinking had on performance—it pulled you out of it. When you play a piece of music, thinking always lags behind what is happening, so you get further and further behind where the piece actually is until it all grinds to a halt. The art of performance is to do all the thinking and analysing while practising, so that during the concert you can trust your senses—just listening to the music, feeling the sensation of your fingers on the keys, feeling your emotions. It's like watching with an incredible clarity, yet being directly involved, with nothing between you and the music. You *feel* it, not think it.

I started to compare this experience with my meditations and realised that the reason I and other musicians were prepared to put so much effort into our art, was that it brought us to this wonderful state of complete absorption in what we were doing. It's a vibrant state: clear, totally alive and rich with feeling—and this is communicated to an audience in the best performances of music.

I realised that music and meditation were the same; the only problem was that musicians didn't know it. They didn't derive the benefits of meditation because this wonderful state only happened while they were actually performing—as soon as the concert stopped, it stopped too.

Meditation allowed me to enter this absorbed state whenever I wanted to. It didn't require expensive equipment or elaborate preparations—it just meant doing the meditation exercise.

Battling with the big questions

The background to this was Australia where I studied music and education; on completion of my studies I was extremely fortunate to win a scholarship to study in Paris. For three years I worked with the composer Olivier Messiaen, who was one of the great French composers of the last century, and his wife, the pianist, Yvonne Loriod.

While in Australia I battled with all the big questions. Under the guidance of a psychiatrist friend I studied Freud and Jung extensively and received a fairly thorough dose of psychotherapy. With a philosopher friend I gained an understanding of the principles of philosophy and logic and read the major philosophers of the West. This all fed into my doctoral thesis on Messiaen's music, which covered the major art movements and formative ideas of the 20th century as he was strongly influenced by these (as were nearly all his contemporaries).

So, in one sense I arrived in Paris thoroughly prepared, and in another, with a lot of baggage. What amazed me was that all this work and my fortunate position didn't make the slightest bit of difference to how I felt. Although my teachers became friends and, as is the tradition in France, took me in as a son and I lived in a protected world, the boundaries of this world seethed with jealousy and rivalry the same as anywhere else, only on a much larger scale.

I found I wasn't exempt from any of these emotions and whether I liked it or not, was ranged on one side of one of the great musical wars of French cultural life. My tongue could be as critical and cutting as anyone else's. I had hoped that somewhere would be free from war. This was where the penny dropped that I was wrong. Or rather, as I found through opening up to the meditation path, I wasn't completely wrong—I was just looking in the wrong place.

Jumping in

The next step on my path to discovering the meditation tradition was being invited to go to Antwerp with my Canadian friend to meet his teacher, who was also Canadian. Apparently this teacher had trained in a Burmese monastery and was subsequently recognised by His Holiness the 16th Karmapa (the head of the Kargyu order in Tibet) as a high Tibetan lama.

So I met him but was surprised by his apparent lack of seriousness. In fact, I decided he was a dilettante, as his talks weren't prepared and were quite casual. For example, he once came in announcing that he had forgotten what he was going to say and that this was odd because he had read so many books. This, of course, was not very impressive to someone who identified with being a scholar! However, without knowing it, my dialogue with Namgyal Rinpoche began—I was gently being sent up.

My first real lesson came in Crete, where I attended my first meditation course during a summer holiday on the south coast of the island. My friend, his wife and I travelled by train from Paris to Greece and then caught the ferry to Crete. We arrived to find most people camping and a rather casual, holiday-like atmosphere. I was surprised because I had taken time off from work and saw this as a serious opportunity to understand the meditation tradition.

On the third day, when Namgyal had simply given a talk each morning and afternoon, I felt as though I had wasted my time and made a mistake becoming involved; I was also somewhat insulted by the casualness of it all. After all, I was extremely busy, used to being serious and purposeful and had expected to be set to work. At this particular morning's talk Namgyal casually remarked, "Oh, by the way, the people from Paris, go and have a swim". This was the final insult! However, after an hour or so I calmed down and decided to have a swim.

As I got into the water, which was beautifully warm, a whole new world opened up. I realised I had not been near the sea for over two years, and had never given myself time to actually *feel* the sea. It was a revelation. My skin opened up and the sea soaked in. My eyes opened and I really *saw* the light on the sea and land and the incredible colours of the sea, sky and rocks. I smelt and tasted the air and sea. Although trained as a musician I had never experienced the sound of the sea going right through my body.

And so the world of meditation opened up. I was brought straight out of my highly structured, planned and busy life right into the present moment. I had to admire the timing of the instruction! Namgyal had waited and then caught me perfectly on my serious and intense identity, piercing it skillfully. I realised he knew my mind better than I did, and that I had a lot to learn. I had met a tradition that was profoundly serious but also humorous and playful.

My experience in the sea was the basis of meditation in a nutshell. No books, no thinking, no effort, just naturally opening the senses. Moving the mind from thinking to inner sensing—to the direct experience of our bodies. As I learned later, the reason this had such a profound effect on me was because I was thoroughly prepared and very focused. With perfect timing, Namgyal had taken me out of my comfort zone into a world which I actually *experienced* for the first time.

It was the same lesson I learned at the piano—to go beyond thought. Instead of looking out at the world, seeing what was happening, working it out, seeing it as "out there", I was suddenly in it, and it was in me. The experience was so direct there was no distinction between me and the sea—only the seeing, hearing, tasting, smelling and feeling. There wasn't any me to experience it. It was a real shock; I had been very skillfully led to experience the natural intelligence and awareness of my own body. Of course, at the time, I had no idea what had really happened and no way of explaining it.

Bringing the meditation tradition to the West

So I started to listen more closely to what was being said at the retreat and found that behind the light facade was a profound knowledge and experience of Buddhism. Namgyal was one of the first teachers in the West, along with Chogyam Trungpa in America, to attempt to integrate the practical philosophy of Buddhism with Western life and culture.

He was revolutionary in taking all the latest ideas and movements in the West and relating them to the Eastern tradition of meditation. As I came to understand Buddhism and the practical tradition of meditation, I could see that from this perspective what Namgyal was doing was brilliant. He was stripping Buddhism of all its cultural accretions to reveal the direct, practical experience and knowledge inherent in it, and relating it to experience in Western culture. One of his gifts was his ability to re-translate the original texts by tracking the roots of the Pali words to derive their original meaning and intent.

After the retreat I returned to Paris for my final year of study faced with a difficult decision. In front of me was a wonderful music career; it was suggested I could get a position in Paris, but I could see exactly what I would be doing for the rest of my life. On the other hand I could learn this amazing new discipline, but I knew that if I took it on properly it would cost my music career, because it was essential to move straight into a position after my study was completed. My choice was between continuing to take *my ideas* about my life seriously, or taking *life itself* seriously.

So I sat on this decision, waiting and watching. As the year progressed and I successfully gave my debut recital in Paris, I realised I was going to have to step into the unknown. (My music teachers were naturally upset and puzzled at this decision, but they were very understanding and we have remained friends and kept in contact.)

I then went into retreat in the beautiful town of Assisi in Italy for a year, where learning with Namgyal was a continuation of what I was used to with my music teachers. He set exercises and I would check the results after I completed them. I spent the year studying ancient meditation texts, doing the advanced practices of Insight meditation and the visualisations, mantras and yogas of Tantra.

After this I returned to Australia and took a position at my old university until the Lifeflow Meditation Centre evolved to the point where it demanded most of my time. I also continued my meditation training, which included another two years of retreat, and covered all the different forms of Buddhism: Burmese Insight practice, the original philosophical and psychological texts and teachings, the developments of Tibetan Buddhism with its rich tradition of philosophy, visualisation, mantra and Tantra, and also Zen.

A teaching for our culture

My aim has been to bring the skills and knowledge of the meditation tradition into our own culture so that it can be fresh, up-to-date, and completely free from the jargon, cultural habits and beliefs which come as part of the package.

In the East, the structures and systems of teaching do not provide the means to integrate advanced experiences into our way of life—they rely on a lifestyle that is preordained and usually monastic (and, in fact, many of these advanced experiences open up views not integral to our culture). I realised that the way meditation is taught in the East takes for granted the institutions supporting this meditation work, and these institutions do not exist in our own culture.

Western Buddhist centres, because they see themselves as part of a traditional religion, have largely taken on the forms and structures of religious institutions. By default, they have tended to take on the flavour and forms of Christianity, whether Catholic in the Tibetan centres or Protestant in the others. I much preferred the structures associated with music and universities.

I see no point in struggling with the rules and rituals that are part and parcel of a monastic tradition, which are necessary if you are living in a monastery. Very few of us are doing that. Similarly, it is pointless trying to gain the kinds of results that require the highly specialised lifestyle taken for granted in a monastery. Many teachers forget, or perhaps don't even know, that much of what is taught in meditation exists because in Asia many boys go into monasteries when they are quite young and need to be kept busy. There's a lot of testosterone and no football! The Buddhist tradition is the only training they know—the structures are feudal and the discipline strict.

We, on the other hand, come to meditation with a lot of schooling and possibly university experience behind us—so we know how to concentrate. Meditation can then be used to become aware of what is happening when we are concentrating, and do it much more skillfully, without ignoring our bodies. We can then apply this skill of calm concentration to every part of our lives instead of just in the area of our work.

Lifeflow Meditation

I have aimed to build an Australian form of meditation—being true to the tradition that has been handed on, but adapting it so it works in a democratic, free country where we earn our living, respect each other's individuality and are attempting to overcome the kinds of unfair discrimination that can be ingrained in social habits. My particular focus and interest has been in creating an accessible form of the advanced practices of meditation. These are usually locked in very complex and almost impenetrable structures that render them virtually unintelligible. Of course, some of this has been deliberate because some practices can only be handed on directly, but jargon and obfuscation have always been the tools of specialisation.

I have found this advanced material valuable, interesting and exciting—it is a rich, deep stream of knowledge and experience, and I have sought to stay true to this depth. Much of the material is unique to the Eastern meditation tradition and has never been part of our culture. I would like to see this material integrated into our culture while respecting its value and roots—and I have found it possible to do this. You don't have to learn Tibetan, Pali or Sanskrit or learn a lot of arcane material; most of the latter is cultural and has nothing to do with the original intention of the exercises.

So with the team of teachers in the Lifeflow Meditation Centre, and advice from people experienced in organisational structure, we established a curriculum to supply the necessary groundwork in a structured way. This enables someone who has no previous experience of meditation to attend a course to learn the basics so they can use it as a tool in their lives. If they become interested, or have previous experience, they then have the opportunity to pursue their interest as far as they wish.

Teaching at the Lifeflow Meditation Centre is student-centred and each person is able to proceed at their own pace. The Centre has had a code of ethics in place since its inception, and this has been adapted to give clear guidelines for teaching and provide useful principles for members, which are applicable to everyday life. Membership is optional, and not a prerequisite for attending courses.

Four terms of courses are run each year at our city centre. There are six classes each week of Level 1, which is the basic course where the skills of meditation are taught, three classes each week of Level 2, and one each of Levels 3 and 4. Strong links have been forged between the Centre and psychologists, doctors, therapists and other health professionals and an academy of natural health. Regular retreats are run at our retreat centres, with public retreats spanning weekend retreats to seven-day retreats and members' retreats also ranging from weekends to ten days. (Further information about Lifeflow retreats is provided in Chapter 11.)

Finding a lifestyle

Although I was ordained as a Lama in the Karma Kargyu lineage of Tibetan Buddhism by His Holiness the Karmapa many years ago, the Karmapa understood that I was going to have to experiment to integrate the meditation tradition with my own culture, and supported my work of adapting the practices and developing a way of life which would suit me as an Australian. I have therefore never worn robes or used a Tibetan name and never espoused celibacy. However, I found learning self-containment and how to generate inner ecstasy (from the meditation stream of Tantra) invaluable for developing emotional balance and strength.

I searched for a way to live that embodied the freedom and self-contained quality of the monks I met, while retaining a sense of community and remaining true to being Australian. I knew I wasn't destined to get married and have children because I had been looking for some time for a way to commit myself to the inner life. Yet I didn't want to become a pseudo-Tibetan or be locked up in a feudal system based on rejecting the opposite sex. Originally Buddhist monks were simply called "wanderers" because it was a life based in nature (the monasteries, structures, rules, rituals and beliefs came later) and based on the freedom to question and wander.

By building on the freedoms we have in our culture, the knowledge and experience we have developed in relating to each other, a love of nature, the tradition of music teaching, the intellectual tradition of our university culture, and the principles of the inner life of the East, I have found a way to live that embodies the essence of the original "wanderer". It is a life that fits effortlessly into our culture, where you have the freedom to fully explore and open the inner life, and time to give to teaching and the community.

Freedom from emotional conflict

Through training and insight I came to understand how our experience is filtered through our thoughts, perceptions and memories. We seldom experience our senses directly so are therefore rarely in complete touch with the life around us. Opening our senses to life is one of the easiest things to do because it is completely natural. When our senses are open and we *experience directly*, without thinking about it or trying to interpret it, we make contact with our original mind, the mind without thought.

However, it is almost impossible *not* to interpret what we are experiencing—it is a deeply ingrained habit, because we like to be in control and to know what is happening. This is where the conflict begins and is the war constantly waged in our own hearts. It is the conflict between what our bodies are actually experiencing and how our minds interpret this. Sometimes they work together, but most of the time we choose the memory or story in our minds over resting with the experience of our bodies.

I found it is possible to live without getting caught up in stories and conflicts—but it can only be done when we come to accept ourselves, and know our own minds. Even though it is a simple process, it is something that human beings have to *learn* to do, because we have learned to think. The cost of learning to think is losing touch with our bodies, which costs us our direct sense experience.

The peace meditation provides is not the dead, bodiless, sexless peace we often imagine peace to be. It is a vivid, vital peace—open and in touch with everything. It is a state of love. The mind, instead of being lost in stories, thoughts and memories, is completely in touch with the body, so it is possible to be right there with what is happening all the time, aware and awake—able to rest completely still or move quickly. This kind of peace is like resting in luminous space, what the meditation stream of Tantra calls *clear light*. This luminous space is everywhere and through everything; it is the matrix in which everything rests.

How to use this book

The aim of this book is to provide you with all the material necessary to develop your own meditation practice, from the very beginning right through to the advanced stages. It outlines the basic principles of meditation, what happens when you meditate and the stages you go through, what you can expect as you build a practice and the theory behind it all. It also contains practical instructions for preliminary exercises and the different kinds of meditations, which are clearly marked in boxes so you can easily refer to them.

The book is divided into three parts which are outlined in detail below. Part One contains all the material taught in the introductory (Level 1) course of the Lifeflow Meditation Centre; Parts Two and Three contain the material taught in Levels 2, 3 and 4. The meditations outlined in the book are taught in those meditation courses or in the retreats run by the Centre.

Please take what you find useful for your meditation practice at the moment and leave the rest for later, when it becomes more relevant or you are interested in exploring further.

Part One: **Getting started**

If you are a newcomer to meditation or wish to revise the basics for your practice, Part One provides everything you need to know. It explains how to relax your body and calm your mind quickly and easily in your daily life, how meditation works and the steps of the meditation technique. The deepening stages of meditation are laid out in a simple way so you can recognise them as you meditate.

Part One also introduces all the different kinds of meditations and there are detailed practical instructions for these, and for how to meditate when you are sitting, standing, walking and lying down.

Spot Meditations are also introduced: these short meditations can be done in twenty seconds or less to quickly regain your emotional balance, wherever you are and whatever you are doing.

A chapter is devoted to the Three C Technique, a speciality of the Lifeflow Meditation Centre. This simple technique enables you to apply the awareness gained from meditation to your habits and the situations and aspects of life everyone finds difficult. You will learn how to use this technique to let go of unhealthy and unpleasant emotions, and be introduced to a quick, powerful way of discharging them.

Knowing how your mind and emotions work can take a lot of the mystery and angst out of many emotional states and so this is also explained, demonstrating how meditation can be used as a tool for opening up your intuition and inner world. You will also find many examples of how to use meditation informally in your everyday life.

Finally, there are guidelines for what to expect in a meditation retreat and how to make the most of your retreat experience.

Part Two: Developing a meditation practice

If you are a more experienced meditator who wants to explore the discipline of meditation in detail, you will find in Part Two the material you need to develop your practice.

You will be introduced to the kinds of states that open up as you go deeper into meditation, so you can begin to recognise them and learn to contact them at will. These are commonly called *alternate states, altered states of consciousness or transpersonal states* and they are explained in detail.

Meditation provides the tools to discover how your mind and consciousness actually work, so that you can free yourself from emotional conflict. You can then begin to understand how to use your instinctual energies skillfully and joyfully, which gives you freedom to ride the waves of emotions. In Part Two you will be shown how to develop this skill.

You will also learn how to use the Three C Technique to make decisions—this can be particularly useful when you are faced with making important, potentially life-changing choices.

Using meditation to develop awareness is explained further in Part Two and you will be introduced to meditating on space.

Also included in Part Two are instructions for doing advanced retreats. You will learn how to use retreat to observe how your emotions work and how to free yourself from emotional conflicts. Finally, there are detailed instructions on how to fine-tune your meditation practice.

Part Three: The theory behind the practice

Part Three is for readers who have already developed a meditation practice and who would like to discover what makes meditation tick—the theory supporting the practice. It explores the philosophy and psychology of meditation, from both Western and Eastern cultural perspectives.

Knowledge from both cultures about the brain, mind and meditation is integrated to give you a clear understanding of how meditation can be applied. In Part Three you will discover how to harmonise the way you live with the way your brain and body operate, so that you can work with them rather than fighting against them.

Because it's as easy to get lost in the inner life as it is in the Australian outback, maps are very important. With the correct maps, the journey can be exhilarating and liberating. Part Three provides both Western and Eastern maps of the mind to help you orient yourself and understand how your consciousness works.

You will learn how people tend to orient themselves differently according to personality type, which meditations suit these personality types and how far the different kinds of meditation will take you. You will also be introduced to the different meditation paths that can be followed.

The different streams of the meditation tradition are also explained. You will discover the different skills these streams develop, why they exist in the first place and how to integrate what you have learned into your everyday life.

Introduction

*Being still and open is the blissful state in which
we feel totally at peace with ourselves and the world.*

Meditation is something we could all do naturally and easily as
children—we just didn't know what we were doing. If you observe
a child watching something, completely absorbed, you see how
still they become, how totally open and receptive they are, how
concentrated their mind is and how comfortable they are in their
body. The price of learning to think is that we lose this ability; in fact,
it is often actively discouraged. I remember being told off as a child
for daydreaming when I became completely absorbed in something.
My parents were always telling me that I'd lose my head if it wasn't
screwed on!

The reason for losing this ability is that we can't think and be in touch
with our bodies at the same time. In fact, we spend surprisingly little
of our waking lives in touch with our senses. Yet resting in the senses,
receptive and aware, just taking in everything around us, is the natural
state of our minds and bodies. Being still and open is a blissful state in
which we feel completely at peace with ourselves and the world.

Meditation provides the means to consciously reintegrate the ability
to become absorbed, while maintaining the skills of thinking.

The four streams of meditation

The meditation tradition has developed four distinct streams: **Calm
and Concentration**, **Insight**, **Tantra** and **Ethics**. These have been
developed because meditation is a tool that can be used in different
ways to achieve different purposes. However, no matter what you are
aiming for in meditation, everything rests on the calm, concentration
and balance of the absorbed state, so this is where all meditation
begins.

The stream of Calm and Concentration develops the skills of
meditating, relaxing the body and calming the mind. It outlines how to
deal with thoughts, keeping them in perspective so they do not drive
us, and opens up the deep peace you experience when your mind and
body are balanced and still.

The stream of Insight is a body of knowledge and practice for learning how to see clearly what is happening in our lives, how our consciousness and thought processes actually work, and how to avoid being caught in our emotions.

The stream of Tantra provides exercises for learning how to keep our emotions in a healthy state, so we can create good feelings for ourselves and learn to sustain them. This stream also allows us to come to know the naturally blissful state of our bodies, to understand our raw instincts and learn how to integrate and use them skillfully rather than being driven by them.

Finally, the stream of Ethics provides a way to apply the calm, clarity and emotional skill of meditation to our everyday actions. It opens up the possibility of basing what we do in our lives, and how we move our bodies through the world, on seeing clearly and responding directly to what happens, free from emotional conflict and ingrained habits. (These four streams are explained in more detail in Chapter 24.)

This book focuses on the stream of Calm and Concentration and is the first in a series of books dedicated to each stream of the meditation tradition. It explains how to balance your mind and emotions and maintain them in a healthy state. It also explores the advanced stages in Calm and Concentration and how to apply those skills to everyday life, to making major decisions and to studying and understanding emotions.

Meditation is a tool

Meditation is a tool for training the mind so that you can use it skillfully, creatively and productively and avoid being caught in the emotional traps which prevent us from living happy and useful lives. Meditation is learned in the same way you would learn a sport, craft, to play a musical instrument or to take up a discipline like science. You need to be guided skillfully by someone who has mastered it, and the more you are able to include it in your life, preferably as a regular practice, the more you progress.

Just sitting down to meditate doesn't mean you will automatically reach a good state. Meditation is only a *tool* to achieve this and like any tool its use needs to be learned properly. I have met many people who have struggled for years with meditation, finding it very difficult or even impossible to meditate—often they assumed, or were told, that it was difficult. They were surprised to discover how simple it actually is when learned properly and, without exception, have been able to relate it to past experiences in their own lives.

For example, one woman remembered that she used to sit on the roof of a shed on the farm where she lived as a child. She loved doing this because she felt close to the sky and could see all around her. She would stay there for ages, feeling peaceful, still, in touch with everything around her and completely content. It was only when she experienced this same state in meditation that she recalled doing it as a child.

Maintaining your emotional health

Meditation brings your mind and body together so they work in harmony, with thoughts and actions supporting each other instead of being in conflict. In meditation practice you learn to achieve your balance—physically, emotionally and mentally—whenever you choose, and to rest in the core of your being. This is a state of "keeping your cool", no matter where you are or what you are doing. You learn to understand your emotions and in particular, to avoid being caught in unhealthy emotions. Ultimately the aim is to be able to maintain your own mental and emotional health.

Since the Second World War, and the general prosperity the West has enjoyed, people have discovered that material wealth does not automatically lead to feeling good or happy. The upsurge in personal development and self-improvement, psychotherapy and self-help books bears witness to this, and they all rest on the promise of feeling better. However, everything that is self-focused is ultimately limited.

This is where meditation comes into its own because it is based on the understanding that our identity and sense of self *is a product of how we think*, so trying to feel better through thoughts doesn't work––being caught in thought itself is the problem. We forget, or didn't ever notice, that feeling good is a *feeling*. It's based in our bodies, not in our heads. Meditation takes you out of thoughts, out of the self, into a wider, deeper view: the world of the body and senses.

Meditation is used to rekindle the ability we had as children to become absorbed in our sense experience. This is the natural, blissful state of our bodies, and in the Zen tradition it is called our *natural mind*, or *original mind*. Meditation, therefore, is used to rediscover the mind we had before we learned to think. We can do this while maintaining and enhancing our thinking skills for two reasons: firstly because we can then become *aware* of our direct sense perceptions (as children we were not aware of what we were doing) and secondly, because when we know what it is like when we are *not* thinking, we can be aware when we *are* thinking, and instead of being lost in thought we can use it. Thinking becomes a skill that serves us well.

So meditation is an invitation to come home to the rich world of our senses. It's a simple thing to do and easy to learn, but the effects can be profound and blissful.

The philosophical questions

Many people come to meditation with questions. These range from personal questions about health to philosophical questions they have been thinking, talking and reading about for years. For example, I was brought face to face with the fundamental questions about our lives in my teens. What makes us do what we do? Where does ambition come from? What drives us? Is it simply a need for love and approval? Where do emotions come from? Who are we trying to please and impress?

With meditation, you can observe your own mind, emotions, thoughts, reactions and mental processes. You can also study consciousness itself and the whole process of thought. Questions that philosophers, scientists and psychologists are still battling with were explored and answered in the meditation tradition thousands of years ago. The Eastern tradition has mapped this territory thoroughly and Western psychologists are now finding the insights and methods of this tradition extremely valuable in their own work. (My earlier book *Insight and Love*[1] is dedicated to the stream of Insight and to exploring the fundamental questions.)

When you begin to meditate you find that your mind becomes clear and alert—this kind of clarity is a natural consequence of an absorbed state of mind, which you learn in the stream of Calm and Concentration. As you learn to sustain this, you can become aware of things and points of view you normally would not notice. This quality of awareness allows you to see clearly into the habits, situations, emotions and assumptions of your own life. As you develop this awareness in your meditation, insights can naturally occur which enable you to change those habits and assumptions.

The answers or insights into fundamental questions gained through meditation practice have a direct effect on how we see ourselves, our lives, life itself and our place in the universe. These are not theoretical answers—ideas and thoughts that are interesting for a while but don't actually affect your feelings and habits—but direct experiences that completely penetrate your mind and body. Your body and your own experience are an integral part of the answer.

Part One: Getting started

Chapter 1: Setting the scene: what is meditation?

> *Mind training takes into account everything we experience, from the sensations and feelings of our bodies to the undercurrent of emotions and thoughts that run our lives.*

The English word *meditate* means to think about something deeply or to reflect on something. It originally comes from the Latin word *meditari*, which means "to reflect upon". If you did any kind of meditation in the Western tradition up until quite recently, you would have been given a theme or text to meditate on (to think about). If you were in holy orders, or even if you went to do a short retreat, all your meditation would be concerned with reflecting on ideas, prayers, verses and so on. So meditation has always been equated with thinking.

However, in the East, reflecting on ideas is only one form of meditation—there are many others (and they are all explored in this book). Therefore, *meditation* is not really the right word for this Eastern practice but it is the closest and most popular term for describing it. Meditation in the Eastern tradition is something quite new to our contemporary culture (although there were similar practices in the West during the Middle Ages).

The original meaning of meditation in the Eastern tradition is "mind training" or "mental development". Mind training has nothing to do with either thinking about things or the vague, fuzzy state you might get into when you first set out to meditate. These are the two states of mind our culture is very familiar with and which we tend to take for granted. We're either thinking and working hard, being sharp, planning and remembering, *or* we're switched off and fuzzy or asleep—slightly comatose.

From a very early age in our culture we're taught to look after our bodies. We feed, wash and clothe ourselves each day to maintain our physical health and we know that exercise is good for us. Most of us have spent at least ten years at school gathering knowledge and learning to think, so we also have a certain amount of mental training.

What about feelings? What training do we get emotionally? Every time I ask a student or client this question I invariably see a puzzled look until they realise that we don't actually get any. One teenage boy answered this question very succinctly when he said, "You wing it!" It is left to chance and to what we pick up from our own parents' behaviour and habits.

We also take for granted the idea that emotions are personal, involuntary, vague and caused by what happens around us or other people. However, in the East (for example, Tibetan culture) emotional knowledge and training has been developed to the same degree the West has developed physical, technological and scientific knowledge.

Meditation, in its original sense of *mind training*, takes into account everything we experience, from the sensations and feelings of our bodies to the undercurrent of emotions and thoughts that run our lives. It is possible to train our emotions and thought processes, to learn how to use them extremely skillfully and provide the basis for a happy, productive life. None of it has to be left to chance.

This chapter explores the basics of meditation, explaining how it actually works and what effect it can have.

What does meditation do?

Putting it simply, meditation is a tool for developing and maintaining mental and emotional health. We have much more control over this than we realise, and learning how to use meditation can save us from many of the problems that have become endemic and which are totally preventable.

Our mental and emotional health can also have a profound effect on our physical health. Dr Andrew Weill , in his book *Spontaneous Healing*, says: "All illnesses should be assumed to be stress-related until proved otherwise. Even if stress is not the primary cause of illness, it is frequently an aggravating factor[2]." I would add that the same applies to nearly all the common psychological problems which have become so prevalent.

Meditation moves the focus of your mind from your thoughts to your senses; from the endless conversation in your head—the plans, hopes, worries and fears—to your body and what you are actually experiencing. With meditation you can become aware of how your thoughts and emotions operate, see where they come from, how they relate to each other, and how they affect your body and your life, and learn to work with them with a great deal of precision.

Like all tools, meditation can be used skillfully or unskillfully depending on how well you learn to use it. A meditation teacher is exactly like a sports coach, mentor, or music teacher; you would take for granted having tennis or music lessons if you wanted to learn these skills. While you could eventually learn them by yourself, it would be a rather long and inefficient process. As human beings we learn best through imitation, by engaging our bodies, through watching and feeling what it is like when someone who knows how to do something shows us.

In summary, meditation is a tool for doing three things:

1. maintaining your mental and emotional health by knowing how to calm and balance your emotions whenever you choose. By moving the focus of your mind from your thoughts to your senses you literally "come to your senses" and re-establish contact with your body. This brings your mind, body and emotions into alignment so they feel completely connected and balanced.

2. developing the clarity of *mindfulness* and *awareness*. When your thoughts are connected with your body—with what you are doing and feeling—you are *mindful* of what is happening. Your thinking is focused on your sense experience and as you rest with this, your sense *awareness* opens up. Your senses are always aware, and you experience this without any thinking at all. As you open up to your inner sensations you also open your awareness to the world around you, because your sensations are the gateway to both your inner life and the outer world.

3. exploring your inner life. As you rest with the inner sensory experience of your body, you open up the world of your inner experience. Your body registers everything that happens and has ever happened in your life. In meditation it is perfectly safe to open up to all this information. And, of course, it doesn't stop with your personal experience. Your body is the repository of the coded, genetic information that is handed on from generation to generation, and so is the storehouse of all human experience. This is the world of your intuition.

Finding and maintaining balance

One of the most wonderful things about meditation is that you discover what it feels like when your body, emotions and mind are simultaneously balanced, which is an extremely blissful state to be in. It is the resting point of our lives, the space of deepest relaxation and maximum potential, both still and dynamic—an alert, clear and calm state from which it is possible to move in any direction. It is relaxed and poised, with all the senses alive and open.

Achieving this calm state of mind is the basis of all meditation practice. It is not necessarily an end in itself, but it is essential for training our minds. So it's the place where all practice begins and the majority of meditation exercises exist for the purpose of bringing the mind to a calm and concentrated state.

The mind has two qualities—it can move and it can be still. When the mind is moving it scans different objects and thoughts, moving from one to another. When the mind is still it is open to everything. The way you bring the mind to stillness is to focus on a meditation object. It's not the object itself which is important—just the fact that it serves as a single focus point on which your mind can rest. Naturally the mind moves away, but as you keep bringing it back, it gradually becomes calmer and calmer and eventually stays with the object and becomes still. It's rather like training a puppy to sit—it keeps getting up, running away, looking for attention, but gradually learns to stay in one place.

As the mind becomes stiller, the object of meditation becomes less and less important and the mind opens to its natural, fundamental state of just being aware, without being aware of anything in particular. This is the stable core of our minds—the foundation of the mind—and is the great discovery of the meditation tradition. All meditation experience, inquiry and discovery are built on this foundation. It has many names—the *heart of awakening, the mind of awakening, the ground of being, the core of our being, the natural mind*. It is a clear, open, vibrant, spacious stillness, beyond separation and differentiation.

The still mind, the core of our being, is constant and unchanging. You touch it every time you meditate. In this state, because you are not focused on anything in particular, you are aware of your *whole* body, instead of just a part of it, and you are also aware of everything around you. You are simply resting in awareness.

This stillness is the state in which you are completely balanced. The aim of meditations that focus the mind to bring it to a calm and concentrated state, is to enable you to find this balance point whenever you want, and learn to hold it.

The space between the thoughts

From this point of stillness you can learn to stay aware and just watch. It's not an escape but a place of clarity. Discovering the mind when it is still is like discovering that clouds are not the only things in the sky. In fact, it's like discovering the sky itself—vast, luminous and clear. As you recognise this foundation state of the mind, you can rest there as thoughts and emotions move through your mind and body, like clouds in the sky.

You can then *see* them—moving in a stream, coming and going—instead of being caught in them. Thoughts and emotions themselves don't cause problems for us, any more than clouds in the sky cause problems. It's *not seeing the context in which they operate and how they work* that causes our problems. It's also clinging to them and thinking that they are all that exists in the mind.

As you learn to let them go you don't become feelingless, as some people fear. You actually develop the confidence to feel more, to completely open to your feelings, because thoughts and emotions lose their power over you. You begin to understand how they work and either ride them with confidence or let them go.

Accepting thoughts and emotions as they are, giving them the space to be, and learning to watch them instead of being caught in them means you become freer in your emotional life, because you don't feel that controlling or manipulating thoughts and emotions is the only way you can relate to them.

Finding the "beach" and learning to float in the "sea"

I like to use the sea as a symbol for the mind for two reasons: it is used throughout the history of the meditation tradition and in Australia all of our major cities are on the coast so many of us love the sea.

When we learn to swim, we need to know that the sea exists, its different moods, waves and currents and where the beach is. The mind is like the sea in that it has moods, waves, rips and currents. Yet many of us treat our mind incredibly casually, ignoring its different moods and states, getting caught in them, and then wondering what is happening. Occasionally we experience a moment of calm when the waves go still, before another storm comes along and we are picked up and thrown from one wave to the next and eventually dumped.

As with swimming there needs to be a reference point from which we can start in meditation, so we need to know that we can get out of the "sea" and find the "beach". Developing calm and concentration in meditation is like finding the beach—finding the place where the mind is still and we are safe. The next step is learning to float, and this describes what it feels like as we begin to meditate.

When learning to swim, we start by going into the sea where it is shallow and calm so we can learn not to fight and can then take the step of letting our feet leave the ground. We discover that the sea will hold us. It's exactly the same in meditation. Having established that there is a place where the mind is still and calm (the "beach") we can, by learning to let go, take the step of learning to float—to rest the mind in our sense experience. In the same way we discovered the sea will hold us when we learn to let go and float, we discover that the sensations we are focused on hold our mind when we let go of our thoughts.

Dealing with thoughts—the waves on the ocean

In the next stage we learn how to deal with thoughts. Thoughts are exactly like waves on the ocean. If we get caught in them they will drive us and the only choice we then have is to wait until they break. In the beginning of establishing calm and concentration, it is crucial to know how not to get caught in thoughts and the technique is exactly the same as a surfer uses. By studying waves and knowing the ocean when it is calm, a surfer sees waves before they arrive and can then decide whether to ride them or not. If a wave is not good to ride, a surfer will dive under it, knowing that the ocean under the wave is relatively still. The wave then goes over the top.

Meditating is the same. If a thought comes along that is going to disturb the meditation, the technique is to let the thought go into the background and bring your mind back to the meditation object. This allows you to keep calm and "dive underneath" thoughts—you will then see them coming, notice them, and just let them ride over the top without catching you.

Many people are led to believe that meditating means having no thoughts in the mind at all. So they spend their meditation trying not to think and find this is impossible—it just gets worse! Trying to stop thoughts is exactly like trying to stop waves on the ocean. Thoughts are a natural part of the mind. The technique is to learn how to deal with them, which means accepting them and seeing them before they hit, like waves on the ocean, so we can dive under them.

Moving from a point of balance

Meditation allows us to maintain our mental and emotional balance so that when we move or make decisions, we are moving from a point of balance. As with any physical activity, if you move from a balanced state, the resulting movement will be skillful and effective. And if you are not balanced when you move, then you get further and further out of balance and so eventually fall over. This explains why good intentions often go astray. We have all been in situations where we were genuinely trying to help, but find ourselves caught in the emotional storm just like everyone else.

Decisions are the beginning of actions, and learning to make decisions from this point of balance is a way to ensure that the actions arising from our decisions will also be skillful and effective. I discuss this in detail in Chapter 14.

The next chapter explores meditative concentration and how you can find space and time for meditation in your life.

Chapter 2: **Beginning to meditate**

Finding a suitable time and place you can keep for meditation is the best way to keep it going.

This chapter explores all the practicalities of beginning to meditate, starting with what concentration means in meditation and how it differs from our usual idea of concentration. It discusses how to find the time and place to meditate and how to keep clear divisions in your life.

Chapter 2 also explains how to set yourself up for meditation, beginning with very useful physical loosening exercises, and provides instructions for sitting, standing, walking and lying down.

Developing meditative concentration

There is a major difference between meditative concentration and the kind of concentration we were usually forced to do at school. While learning to concentrate as children we were invariably brought to a state where we had to deny our bodies. We were often not calm but under pressure, so controlling the body and forcing ourselves not to feel it became integral to the process. There are few people who associate the word *concentration* with pleasure and this is a real shame, because a truly concentrated state of mind is an extremely pleasurable experience.

The first time I taught meditation to sixty teenaged boys (aged twelve to sixteen) at a private school, they were fairly suspicious and sceptical and, as this was the first time anyone had introduced them to meditation, the teachers were very nervous about the outcome. I explained the process of meditation and said that in meditation, when you learn to concentrate, your body is part of the process. It needs to be in a relaxed state so it feels good, rather than tight and uncomfortable—you don't have to force yourself to concentrate. If you look after the body first, it works with you and supports your mind as it becomes increasingly focused. Well . . . they looked a bit stunned but after loosening up the body we settled down to meditate.

The results were remarkable because during the meditation not one boy moved. After three meditation classes their teacher asked them to comment on the course by writing anonymously five positive and five negative things about the experience. Fifty students said they couldn't find anything negative and those that did said that some of it was a bit boring. One said he'd rather play football. The overwhelming majority liked the experience, finding it extremely relaxing and noting that it improved their concentration markedly at school.

Our culture is not alone in believing that to concentrate, or to train or "purify" the mind you have to punish the body. Asceticism was, and is, just as popular in the East as the West. The Buddha initially gave himself fully to this belief. After an idyllic life of pleasure, sport and study where, as a prince, nothing was denied him, at the age of 29 he took up the life of an ascetic to "purify" his mind. One of his major discoveries was that asceticism made no difference. He found that neither indulging the body nor denying it gave any insight into how the mind, emotions and body worked, and both left you trapped in the undercurrent of thoughts and emotions. Hedonism and asceticism are two sides of the same coin—trying to deny the reality of the body by denying the existence of pain (hedonism) or by denying the existence of pleasure (asceticism). So he accepted his body, had a good meal, made himself comfortable and his mind opened clearly.

Looking after the body is essential to concentration. The Buddha called this "the middle way". It's a state in which the body, emotions and mind are balanced, because they are all being accepted. It's the *natural* state of the mind and body, which is blissful, peaceful and nourishing, and this is the hallmark of meditation.

Finding the time and place

For those people who are just beginning to meditate, finding a time and place takes a conscious effort. Many people find it very difficult to keep clear divisions in their lives—between work and home, day and night, between each week, and each task at work. Things tend to run into each other and there is no relief from constant pressure. Meditation allows you to become aware of this, and to consciously build these divisions into your life.

One of the main skills you acquire from learning to balance yourself mentally and emotionally is beginning to feel the cycles of your mind and body (I discuss this in detail in Chapter 9). Catching and using one of the natural cycles of your body and the day is the best way to establish a regular time and place for meditation. Your mind and body will get used to it and automatically respond just by being there.

So if you like the early morning, keep some of that time for your own mental and emotional health by meditating before you start to get busy. Others like the evening, that time between finishing work and going home. And others find the middle of the day works best for them, so take some time off in the office or go outside for a while.

Using the same chair or same place also makes meditation much easier. I always set aside a particular chair to meditate on wherever I am staying because I find that as soon as I sit down my body responds. It doesn't matter whether your place is in the house or garden, in the car or at work, as long as it can become a habit.

Those who find it difficult to meditate at home have found that meditating in the car, before driving off to work or when arriving at work, and again when coming home and parking in the carport, works very well. A number of people have found a car park by the sea or a nature reserve, where they can meditate comfortably for five to ten minutes. (See also Chapter 10 on informal meditations, for more ideas about how to incorporate meditation into your life.)

Some people get quite inventive and find that the things they were worried about—perhaps the dog or cat or even a young child—turn out not to be a problem at all. One student had a large Alsatian dog who would howl outside the door whenever he tried to meditate. So eventually he gave up and opened the door; from then on there was silence. The dog would happily rest its head in his lap and stay there for the entire meditation period.

As you build a meditation practice, finding a suitable time and place you can *keep* for meditation is the best way to keep it going. Let it become a habit, like cleaning your teeth or having breakfast. Don't get too fussy with this—just see what works. Meditation can then take its place in your daily life, just like having a shower. In fact, this is the best way to view meditation—it does for your mind and emotions exactly what a shower does for your body.

Let the people you live with know what you are doing so they get used to it—you can explain that it's just like having a shower. And let the answering machine or message bank look after the phone. Remind yourself that your mental and emotional health is important and that you will deal with things much more effectively when you are in a clear, calm state.

Keeping clear divisions

Being balanced depends on being able to make and keep clear divisions—both in meditation and in life. Our minds and bodies naturally seek to complete each action before moving onto the next.

I think one of the major problems in workplaces is that no job is ever completed before the next one starts. They then pile up in the mind, without end. There's not much any of us can do about this, even if we own the company. However, there's a lot we can do for our minds and bodies. If you do a very short meditation (see Chapter 6: Spot Meditations) before moving from one job to another, you allow your mind and body to let go of the previous job and prepare for a new one. This makes a clear division between the jobs, and your mind and body can start afresh. Similarly, a short meditation before going to work can prepare you for the day, and another short meditation when work is finished, or when you have just got home, clearly separates your work from home.

Our bodies naturally seek a rest in the early afternoon, so a short meditation during the lunch break takes advantage of this and restores your energies for the afternoon. A short meditation before going to bed can prepare you for sleep, because it makes a clear division between day and night. However, I recommend keeping it fairly short, as a long meditation can recharge your energies and so keep you awake.

A young student at a Level 1 meditation course worked as a packer in a supermarket. He had been to the doctor because he was having health problems. The major problem, as he described it, was that he never had a chance to rest or let go—he never finished a job properly because something was always added to what he was already doing.

So he decided to do a Spot Meditation each time he was told to move from one thing to another—a quick Instant Calm Breath, taking a breath right into his belly and letting it out with a big sigh (see Chapter 6). This worked wonders. As I got to know him, I discovered that he and his wife had been unable to have children and were about to start the IVF program. They didn't need to as she became pregnant while he was doing the meditation course!

The same thing applies to people who work with clients. Doing a short Spot Meditation between clients can make all the difference to keeping yourself in a good state. You can look after your mind and body, and give them the cue they need to let go, restore themselves and then move on.

Length and frequency

Initially, ten minutes per day is sufficient to establish your practice. This is plenty of time to build it into your life as a habit and, for most people, will provide the benefits you are looking for. If you want to develop your practice further then the time can gradually be increased to half an hour per session and eventually to one hour, which is the maximum time given to any session of meditation as our natural concentration span is about fifty minutes.

It is very important that you don't try to force your meditation or push the time of the session beyond where it is comfortable. I like to quote a sixteenth century Tibetan abbot who said that short, frequent sessions are far more effective than pushing to do long ones. In this way you stay fresh and alert, maintain your interest, enjoy it and it's easy to do.

Your body will tell you when you've had enough, and listening to your body is much more important than trying to force or control it. Gradually you will find that the sessions naturally become longer. Students in meditation courses are often very surprised to find that as the course progresses, their concentration span and meditation times increase without them even noticing.

It's also a good idea to have one day per week where you don't do any formal practice. This keeps the spontaneity there and allows time for informal meditations (see Chapter 10). It keeps your practice fresh and often meditation experiences occur during these times—it's as though things come to you when you give up looking for them.

A good basic practice can be maintained easily and effectively by doing a 10-minute formal meditation five or six times per week, using a Spot Meditation regularly during the day, and doing one or two informal meditations per week. We'll look at Spot Meditations and informal meditations in Chapters 6 and 10 respectively.

Loosening up

I always recommend to clients and students that they do some physical loosening exercises before meditating to help the body relax and let go of tension. We can learn a lot from animals on this—if you have a pet dog or cat, watch what they do before they lie down to relax or sleep. You will notice they never just plonk themselves down.

A dog will find a spot then go round and round it, checking it out, preparing itself, and then eventually lie down. A cat will also check things out carefully, stretch and possibly paw the ground or carpet a little before lying down. Then they completely relax, and you can feel how soft and pliable the muscles of a sleeping dog or cat become. It's this state of total relaxation that provides the energy for them to be alert and move quickly when they have to. Humans, on the other hand, never completely relax even when asleep; our bodies retain tension and we are still thinking. So instead of being right there when we need to be, often we have to wind ourselves up to generate enough energy.

Most of the problems people have when beginning to meditate come from holding tension in their bodies. The meditation causes them to become aware of this—and feel it. I think it is more effective to take this into account before meditating and include a minute or two of loosening exercises before sitting down to meditate.

Instructions for loosening exercises

Here are some very simple and effective exercises for loosening up your body, which take only a few minutes to do. Adjust them to suit your physical condition.

1. Shaking out the body
Start with your left foot, shaking it to loosen it as much as possible.
Then shake your left leg so that you can feel the calf and thigh muscles loosening.
Shake out the right foot, calf, and thigh.
Then shake both hands and arms to loosen them.
Then give your whole body a shake.
Finish by giving your whole body a good stretch.

2. Loosening the shoulders

Rotate each shoulder three times, forwards and backwards. Do this slowly and deliberately so that you feel the physical sensation of moving your shoulders.

Then rotate them together three times, forwards and backwards.

3. Shoulders and neck

Breathe in and pull your shoulders up tightly, deliberately tensing the shoulder muscles.

Then take them back and hold them there for a little while.

While breathing out, let them down slowly.

(This is a good exercise to do every hour or during the day to alleviate the build up of tension in the shoulders.)

4. Neck stretch and massage

Link the fingers of both hands.

Then place them on the back of your head.

Drop your head forward.

Use the weight of your hanging arms to gently stretch the back of your neck.

Hold this position for a little while.

Then bring your head up to loosen your neck muscles, but leave your hands in position, and you will find that your thumbs are in the right position to massage the back of your neck.

5. Neck massage

Using one hand, grip the back of your neck with the heel of the palm and the fingers of your hand.

Massage into the neck, feeling deeply into the muscles.

(This is a good exercise to use often during the day, especially when getting out of a chair or when seated for a long time. You can do it in front of others without them noticing what you are doing.)

6. Swinging from side to side

Stand with your feet about shoulder-width apart, your knees very slightly bent, and swing your body from side to side.

Let your arms swing loosely so it feels as though they are pulling your body with them.

This exercise massages the muscles on either side of the spine and helps to balance your body.

7. Yoga massage

Make a fist with your left hand.

Gently tap your chest repeatedly, so your fist is bouncing lightly on your chest, just above the sternum. (According to the yoga tradition, tapping lightly on your chest, just above the sternum, stimulates the immune system.)

Then tap lightly down the inside of your right arm and up the outside.

Repeat this process with your right hand so that you massage your left arm.

Tap all over the front of your body with both hands, then the small of the back, the backside and the legs.

Then with the tips of your fingers tap all over the back of the neck and the head.

Posture

Because balance is the key, I don't like to be too demanding when it comes to posture for meditation. In the East the prescribed postures, which are usually quite detailed, assume a protected, undemanding way of life because the meditation tradition developed in monasteries where the obstacles to meditating were virtually the opposite of what we face.

Having a protected and specialised life meant that the greatest obstacle to concentration was being too relaxed and having little to do! If you are young and healthy, with no opportunity to play sport, living under extremely strict rules, studying, chanting and meditating most of the day, you need to push yourself and be kept in a taut, alert state. A whack on the shoulders every so often with a stick adds a little excitement to the day! Under those conditions, a posture and discipline that kept a large degree of tension to keep the mind focused were essential.

However, modern life tends to be stressful, and often the tension in our body has become so chronic and habitual that we don't even notice it. If, when we come to meditate, we try to force ourselves into a posture that increases tension and creates pain we will do what we learned at school. We will either try to ignore the pain and push on regardless, aiming to get a good result, or we will give up altogether.

Either way, we have totally undermined the fundamental principle of all meditation, which is to allow the body to relax and the mind to be receptive, to open up to the senses and become aware, without having to censor any of our experience. Naturally, if our bodies are tense, rigid and in pain, this is what the mind will focus on, and then we have a battle to keep it on the meditation object.

As in all things, concentration requires a reasonably balanced state physically and mentally. We need a certain amount of tension, but this needs to be grounded in a relaxed physical and emotional state so that the mind and body are working together rather than in conflict.

Instructions for sitting

On a chair

In the East everyone is used to sitting on the floor; they have been doing it since they were children, so it is a completely natural and relaxed posture. I agree with those who think it is better for the body, but as we are used to sitting in chairs I think this is the best place to begin.

It's best to have a chair that will hold your back reasonably erect, so you are not leaning backwards or forwards. There are many comfortable padded chairs that will provide this support.

Check that your feet are flat on the floor and that your knees are roughly at right angles and well apart to give you a feeling of stability. If the chair is too high for your feet to comfortably rest on the floor, put a cushion under your feet to stabilise them.

Make sure that your backside is well back in the chair.

Place your hands either on your thighs, or together in your lap. (Different meditation schools will give different instructions as to which hand is on top, but there is no need to be fussy, whichever feels most comfortable is the best.)

Hold your neck reasonably straight so that your head feels suspended, as though it is being held up by a string.

On a cushion

For sitting on a cushion, ensure it is high enough to allow your knees to rest on the floor, so that your backside is well off the floor. This provides a strong support for the body; you can then sit erect without having to pull on the back muscles to hold yourself up. Also you won't be leaning backwards, which can often happen if your knees are up in the air.

Sitting on the cushion, you may find it comfortable just crossing your legs, or you might like to place one foot so that the heel is touching the cushion and almost resting in the groin, and putting the other foot in front of it.

If you prefer sitting on the floor but cannot put your knees on the floor, try resting against a wall with a pillow or cushion between your back and the wall. The priority is always that you feel comfortable and your body is being held reasonably erect.

On a stool

If you prefer, you might like to use a meditation stool which enables to you sit comfortably on the floor in a kneeling position. Ensure that your knees are on the floor, back is erect and calves are tucked underneath the stool.

Beginning a meditation

Once you have settled into a good posture, there are three things we teach students to do at the beginning of every meditation. They are *Rocking, Bodycheck, Sounds* and you will find them listed at the beginning of each formal meditation in this book. It is a good routine to establish every time you sit down to meditate as it prepares your mind and body in the best way possible.

Rocking

Rocking from side to side is a very simple way to bring you to your physical balance point and deepen the feeling of balance through your body and mind. It helps you to enter a meditative state quickly as you rock your torso gently from side to side and then let the rocking get smaller and smaller, like a pendulum slowing down. You will find that as you allow yourself to feel this movement, it will eventually stop of its own accord. At this point your body is balanced.

While sitting, gently rock your torso from side to side. Feel the movement along the length of your spine. Just focus on the physical sensations in your body.

As you rock from side to side, allow the movement to get smaller and smaller.

You will find that like a pendulum coming to rest, your body will naturally find its own balance point. Allow your body to gradually become still and rest at that point. Now let your mind open up to this feeling, where your torso is resting at the midway point between your hips.

Now gently rock your head and neck from side to side, again allow this movement to get smaller and smaller until your head gradually comes to rest of its own accord, at the midway point between your shoulders.

Bodycheck

Drop your chin a little to open the back of your neck.

Soften the muscles around your eyes and check that you are looking down very slightly. (Even if your eyes are closed, you might find that you are still staring.)

Check that your jaw and tongue are relaxed and that your teeth are slightly open even if your mouth is closed.

Gently loosen the muscles in your shoulders and abdomen.

Then let a sigh go through your body.

Sounds

When you sit down to meditate there is always noise around you. If you try to insist on perfectly quiet surroundings for your meditation, you will find meditating very difficult. If you allow the sounds around you to be part of your meditation, they will no longer be a disturbance. You can even meditate on traffic noise, and other noises that usually surround us.

Open your mind to all the sounds around you, listening to the sound just as sound.

Listen to all the sounds in the room, in the rest of the building, and all the sounds outside.

Listen all around you.

Listen out as far as you can.

Let yourself be held by the sensation of sound—you might even have a feeling of floating in the sensation of sound.

Then move to the meditation you have chosen.

Moving when you feel the need

As you meditate, don't feel you have to stay perfectly still the whole time. When your body is relaxed and balanced it will make little movements occasionally to adjust itself, and you may feel the need to move slightly. Don't hesitate to do so.

If you need to cough, sneeze or scratch, it is far less distracting for yourself and others (if you are meditating with a group), to simply cough, sneeze or scratch yourself than to try to stop doing it. Just notice what is happening and then return to the meditation object.

Instructions for standing, walking and lying down

Although the meditation tradition developed in monasteries where a lot of sitting meditation was done, it didn't begin there. For most of his teaching life, the Buddha and his followers walked from village to village, living and sleeping outside or in huts. So they developed meditation practices based on standing, walking and lying down as well as sitting; and were expected to be able to meditate in any of these positions. This makes meditation a much more versatile skill!

Standing

For meditating while standing, simply check that your knees are very slightly bent. This is based on the martial arts posture and it automatically brings your body into a balanced position. If you watch a golfer you will see that he or she does exactly the same thing when facing the ball. We are so used to standing with our knees locked and our legs tight that we don't even notice it. This causes a great deal of stress in the muscles in the small of the back.

If you would like to meditate for a longer time while standing, resting your back on a wall is a good way to support yourself. In this position hold your hands together, letting them rest in front of you.

While you are standing and waiting for a bus or a friend is an excellent time to meditate. If you have the kind of job that requires you to be on your feet a lot, such as nursing or working in a store, you don't have to go away to meditate, you can take ten to twenty seconds every so often while you are standing.

Simply bending your knees slightly is enough.

If you have time, then move to your favourite meditation.

Walking

Walking meditation is one of the best ways to incorporate meditation into your life, and there are many exercises you can do. You can just be aware of the movement of your feet as you walk, or you be more controlled about it. For example, one way is to count each step as you walk from 1 to 10 and then back from 10 to 1 again.

Also, while walking, you can easily slip into breathing meditation—just watching and feeling yourself breathing as you walk. You can also bring the steps and your breathing into the same rhythm so that, for example, you breathe in for two steps and breathe out for two.

You can open to the feel of the air on your skin as you walk, noticing how it brushes you, almost stroking you. And you can feel the way your feet touch the earth—letting yourself embrace the earth with your feet (I am indebted to Thich Nhat Hanh for this idea.)

If you are walking in a park or by the sea, listening to the sounds around you—just opening your mind to every sound you hear—can bring you quickly to a meditative state. You can even hear and feel the sensations of the sounds right through your body.

Watching the light on the leaves of trees or looking at colours—just letting your mind rest there as you walk past—is a way to incorporate visual meditations while you walk. (See also Chapter 10.)

To meditate formally while walking, walk slowly in a straight line for about 20 metres or so, holding your hands together either in front of you or behind you, and then turn around and return to your starting point. Repeat this for as long as you feel comfortable.

Lying down

Sometimes you may be too agitated to meditate while sitting, standing or walking, or you may have physical health problems which make it too difficult. Then the easiest way to relax and prepare your body for meditation can be to lie down.

If you are on the floor on a yoga mat, on a bed or in a recliner chair, lie on your back with your hands at your sides or held together on your abdomen. (In this position it is much easier to fall asleep while meditating but it may be exactly what your body needs.)

An alternative posture which is very beneficial for the spine is to bend your knees so that your feet are flat on the floor. Use a reasonably high cushion or pillow under your head. This position supports your spine in its natural curve.

Another more formal posture, which can help keep you alert, is to lie on your side. The right side is usually chosen: place your right hand under your head, keep your knees slightly bent, and place your left hand on your left leg.

Then move to the meditation you have chosen to do (see Chapter 4 for the different types of meditation).

The next chapter outlines the four steps of the meditation technique, which apply to every meditation exercise.

Chapter 3: Developing calm and concentration

There are three qualities which always arise once the mind settles: your body feels relaxed, your emotions become calm, and your mind feels clear.

This chapter explains the four steps of the meditation technique. It also discusses the two ways in which your mind can concentrate and how meditation uses them. The signs of calm and concentration are outlined, so that you can recognise them in your meditations. At the end of the chapter you will find instructions for "tuning" your meditations by becoming aware of how tightly or loosely you are holding yourself.

The meditation technique

When you are developing a state of calm and concentration there are four steps that apply, no matter what kind of meditation exercise you have chosen to do.

1. Relax your body.

2. Focus your mind by allowing it to rest on the meditation object. *This focus is soft, so you are not forcing your mind in any way. Just use the object to give your mind a place to rest.* This opens up your senses and lets thoughts go into the background.

3. When your mind wanders, which it will, just watch where it goes and notice whatever thought or emotion comes along. *This is awareness—it's a receptive process where you open up to the periphery to see where your focus has shifted. This allows you to detach from the thought quickly.*

4. And finally, bring your mind back to the meditation object; use it as an anchor to return to. *Thoughts will automatically arise, and when they do, don't try to get rid of them—just notice them, bring your mind back to rest on the meditation object, and let them go into the background.*

If you find, as your mind naturally wanders through the events of the day and things that are concerning you, that you tend to be caught by a particular thought, a tried and tested method to give yourself some space from it is to name it. So if your work, the conversation you had with your partner or friend, or your plans for the weekend keep catching you, just name whatever it is you are thinking about. This usually allows you to detach from it.

The Buddha outlined the steps of the meditation technique as follows: relax the body (his suggestion was to go into the forest and sit under a tree—more difficult now of course!), slow down the breathing (this enables you to focus on the breath and calm the mind) and let go of whatever comes into the mind (becoming aware of thoughts and emotions and coming back to the breath).

In summary, the four steps for developing calm are:

1. Relax the body.

2. Focus the mind by resting it on a meditation object.

3. Notice thoughts when the mind wanders—just watch them so you are aware of what is happening.

4. Then let thoughts go into the background by gently bringing the mind back to the meditation object.

What kind of meditation object you use to focus your mind depends on the kind of person you are, your background and your lifestyle. For one person, sitting in a chair with their eyes closed and focusing on their breath is the best way to achieve calm, for another a more detailed visualisation exercise works best, and for others a movement meditation is most effective. One of the purposes of formally learning meditation is to find which exercise works best for you.

If you have ever been to a meditation class and been told that there is only one exercise you should do in a certain way with no deviations, then you have had a fairly common experience. However, this is not being true to the meditation tradition. There are actually hundreds of different exercises, with many variations, to suit different types of people and the different ways they experience the world. (Chapter 4 outlines all the different categories of meditation.)

People tend to experience and understand the world in three different ways[3]:

- Some people are visually oriented and think in pictures, preferring to work with images.
- Some are verbally oriented and prefer meditations using sound.
- Others are directly in touch with their bodies so their meditation experience is based on their inner sensations.

You would expect a tradition that understands the human mind to accept this, and it does. So if you prefer one exercise over another or find one much easier to do than others; if you like to sit in a chair or on a stool or on the ground; or even if you prefer your eyes open or shut, it's not a problem. If it is turned into a problem then you are being done a disservice.

Two types of concentration: focused and open

No matter which meditation exercise you choose, you will notice that once you have set yourself up and your body is reasonably relaxed, there are two things you are doing while meditating. You are focusing on the meditation object, and you are also noticing what happens when your mind wanders off to run through its list of things to think about.

These are actually the two types of concentration. The first we are familiar with, because it is taught in school and we use it all the time––*focusing your mind* on something. The second is the ability to open up to a wide view and simply be aware of what is happening. It is a receptive state—you are *open* to whatever comes along.

We are not as familiar with the latter kind of concentration because it is not taught. It is a way to hold your mind still, while opening it to scan everything around you. Both types of concentration are based on the way our brains and senses work. With our eyes for example, we have *focused* vision and *peripheral* vision. This ability also applies to all our senses, so that we can focus on detail when we choose, or open up to the big picture and be receptive to the input of our surroundings.

Indigenous Australians make excellent footballers and have a reputation for having eyes in the back of their heads, because they appear to know exactly where the ball is all the time. I once heard a radio program on which a well-known Aboriginal footballer explained this phenomenon. He said that as a child in northern Australia, he played football late into the evening, even after sunset. Because of this, he developed the ability to *hear* where the ball was. He accessed his *peripheral concentration*, and consciously brought this into the game—a skill which is a natural part of Aboriginal culture.

In meditation you learn how to train both types of concentration.

Training both types of concentration

According to recent research, men generally have a natural ability to focus and women a natural ability to scan. Therefore, the male brain and senses are more attuned to concentrating and focusing on something in particular, while the female brain and senses are more open to the periphery[4].

Men often wonder at the mysterious ability women have to "intuitively" know what someone else is feeling, to find things that have completely disappeared, and to do a number of things at once without seeming to be focused on any one of them. The research shows that women are much more "sensitive" in that they are more attuned and open to the overall input of their senses. This is where their "sixth sense" comes from.

This ability of the senses to open to the periphery is called *awareness* in meditation, and it's just as important as focusing. It is the process of being aware of what your senses are registering without thinking about it. It's a quality of just watching all around, without focusing on anything in particular, and it can be trained.

Learning how to become aware of where your mind has gone when it gets caught by a thought is the only way to free yourself from being taken on a ride. If we are unaware of our thoughts while meditating they keep their power as the undercurrent which runs our lives.

Your mind is naturally moving between focusing and awareness all the time—it focuses on something and then opens to check the surroundings, to see what else might be happening. We are usually conscious of focusing, but don't notice when our minds naturally open up. Therefore, when you follow the four steps of calm, you are training both sides of your mind, both sides of your brain and both sides of your senses. You are focusing, and then when your mind goes off to something else, you open your awareness—move to the periphery, to find out where it has gone.

The signs of calm and concentration—relaxed, calm and clear

Being calm and concentrated is an extremely pleasant state, and there are three qualities which always arise once the mind settles—your body feels **relaxed**, your emotions become **calm**, and your mind feels **clear**.

Of course, this does not happen every time you meditate, as the stresses and strains of every day are different. Sometimes you just need to relax to restore yourself, other times you need to step back from an emotional conflict, or just let your thoughts unwind. However, these are basic things you can check at the end of each meditation to assess how things have gone. This also helps you to recognise and understand what happens as you meditate so that you learn from your own experience and become more skillful in developing your practice.

Your body is relaxed

Firstly, your body feels more relaxed. As the muscles loosen, you become aware of increasingly subtle levels of letting go. You may also become aware of the tightness and discomfort caused by habitual tension in your body.

You will notice your body becoming stiller as it rests more deeply into a state of balance. It may start to feel very heavy as you go deeper into meditation, and at this stage you will find that you cannot physically move. You may recognise it as the same state as when you start to wake in the morning and try to move before your body is fully awake––and find you can't. Alternatively, sometimes as you go deeper into meditation you will find your body becoming very light.

You can also feel warmth and tingling sensations as a feeling of bliss moves through your body and you may also become aware of feeling your *whole* body instead of only parts of it.

You may notice that your senses become more acute as you pick up sounds, smells, tastes, feelings and colours that you normally would not notice. Especially *after* a meditation session, colours are brighter and sounds, smell and tastes are heightened. Your senses are much more open and alert so your sensory experience is more vivid. You may also find that your touch is more acute so that, for example, you become very aware of the contact points of your body with the floor and chair and the feel of your clothes on your skin.

Your emotions are calm

In the same way that your body comes to its natural balance point, your emotions become increasingly still and eventually reach a point of complete calm. This is an inner stillness—a sense of peace and ease as the normal emotional conflicts like worry, busyness, and sense of pressure subside. This can expand to a feeling of being embraced and held by the sense world within and around you, so that you have a feeling of resting or floating in sensations.

Your mind becomes clear

As your senses open your thinking slows down. There will be times when you notice spaces in your meditation—the spaces between thoughts. This can create a feeling of space all around you as your mind lets go of the tight, busy space it normally operates in and opens to both the inner and outer worlds. This sense of spaciousness can be quite luxurious and bring a feeling of relief. From this space you are able to watch everything with a sense of detachment. This is being aware of what is happening but having the space not to become caught in it.

As this space opens you might have inner experiences of light, colour, images and sounds. You might experience heat or cold, and energy moving through your arms, legs and torso. These are all signs that your meditation has gone beyond thought and you have opened to the rich, inner world which is part of our inheritance as human beings.

To summarise, the signs of a calm and concentrated state are:

- Stillness
- Becoming aware of your whole body
- A sense of heaviness or lightness
- Feeling warmth or tingling sensations
- Feeling peaceful and calm
- A sense of space
- Detached watching

You may feel only one of these or a mixture of them—either way it is a clear sign that you are in a balanced state. You will habitually notice one of these more than the others.

After-meditation checklist
After each meditation it's a good idea to run through the following checklist, just to see how it went and to develop the ability to assess your own experience.

- Does your body feel more relaxed?

- Do your emotions feel still and calm?

- Do you have a sense of having more room—of space, of feeling clearer—so that your mind is not so cramped and tight?

These are the three signs of calm and concentration—*relaxed, calm and clear*.

Tuning your meditation
When you get used to meditating you can tune your meditations by becoming aware of how tightly or loosely you are holding your mind and body. It's like learning to tune a musical instrument, and it's amazing how aware you can become of the state of your mind and body while you are meditating.

As you become aware of the habitual places of tension in your body you will find that meditating brings them into sharp focus. This occurs because we all hold our bodies more or less out of balance. This is normal as we are either right or left-handed and so tend to favour one side of our bodies.

As you meditate, your body will naturally find its own balance point. People become alarmed when their head, torso, arms or legs move without their control. And because meditating is like looking through a microscope, the slightest movement, which no-one else would actually see, feels enormous and exaggerated. You can assist this process by understanding what is happening and allowing it to happen, and even encourage it by making the slightest move to find the point where the tension eases.

You can also recognise when you are holding your mind too tightly or too loosely on the meditation object.

Too tight

If your focus is too tight you will become increasingly agitated and find that you are tense and probably trying too hard. In this state, your mind will be jumping around so much that it won't settle down. This is why it is so important to relax your body first, so check that your jaw is relaxed and your shoulders and belly are loose. Check that you are not holding your head too high, as this invariably happens when your focus becomes too tight. In this state you will find that your eyes are staring, even if they are closed, so softening and relaxing them by slightly lowering your gaze will also help.

However, if you find that you are still too agitated, break your session and do something physical—either go for a walk or do the loosening exercises outlined in Chapter 2. Often people find that if they become agitated while meditating, they have forgotten to do some loosening exercises beforehand.

Too loose

If your focus is too loose you will feel a little dull or dazed as your mind drifts off—either to wander all over the place, or to sleep. Your body will slump so a good way to sharpen your concentration is to check your posture, stretch a little and then gently straighten your back. Check also that you have enough fresh air so the room hasn't become too warm or stuffy.

Sometimes you can enter such a deep state of meditation that you don't know what happened and wonder if you fell asleep. It's very easy to check, because if you go to sleep your neck muscles will completely let go and you will find your head slumped on your chest when you wake up again. If your head is reasonably upright, then you didn't go to sleep, no matter what it felt like. And if you do fall asleep, don't worry. It just means your body is tired and needs rest.

Fine-tuning your meditation is discussed in detail in Chapter 18.

The next chapter outlines the seven different categories of meditation and provides practical instructions for all the different meditation exercises—you will be sure to find one that suits you.

Chapter 4: The seven categories of meditation

All meditation exercises, and there are hundreds of them in the Buddhist tradition alone, can be grouped into seven categories.

The seven categories of meditation are: breathing meditation, meditations on inner sensations and energy centres (chakras), visualisation, mantra, movement meditation, contemplative meditation and Insight meditation. The purpose of the first six categories of meditation is to establish calm and clarity, loosen knots in the body and mind (and so heal them), and develop concentration and a state of balance. The reason there is such a large variety of meditations devoted to this is simply because different meditations suit different people. They are all equally effective. The seventh category of Insight meditation is devoted to developing awareness or insight.

This chapter outlines the seven categories in detail and provides practical instructions for the meditations in each category at the end of the chapter.

Breathing

Breathing meditations come in many variations; however, they all fit into two groups—just watching or feeling your breathing, or actually controlling the breath in some way.

Watching or feeling the breath

The simplest, and perhaps oldest form of breathing meditation, is to simply watch or feel the breath at the nostrils, chest or abdomen (depending on which you find more comfortable). You become aware of your breathing, without changing it in any way.

Just watching the breath in this way is one of the most effective ways to quickly reach a state of deep relaxation. It brings you straight into your body, and your thoughts go into the background as you begin to feel the rhythm of your breathing. It is also one of the most useful meditations for overcoming sleep disorders, as it can cut straight through the turbulence of the mind that keeps you awake, and focus you directly and quickly on the natural rhythms of your body.

As you watch your breathing, you will notice its rhythm: quick or slow, shallow or deep, heavy or light, and how long the pauses are between breaths. As you relax and go deeper into meditation, you will notice your breathing becoming slower—each breath becomes longer as the tensions of your body begin to release.

Breathing meditation can bring the mind to a state of profound clarity because it clears the mind of habitual thought patterns to such an extent that you can actually see thoughts come and go. You become aware of the space in which your thoughts operate. You see the spaces between the thoughts and gain a different perspective when you notice that thoughts are only a part of your mind—they are not the whole mind.

Controlled breathing exercises

There are a wide range of meditations based on controlling the breathing, which are used in Yoga (pranayama exercises) and Tantra to bring about certain states. By working consciously with your breath you can create very blissful states, such as a feeling of massaging yourself with the breath. This feeling of massaging your body internally, while floating on the gentle waves of your breath, is one of the most exquisitely blissful meditations. You can develop a sense of it soaking into every part of your body.

Breathing meditation can also create ecstatic bliss as you open to your senses and become receptive to the rich, sensual world of colours, sounds, smells, tastes and feelings, which you can see, hear, smell and feel right through your whole body instead of "out there" where they usually are.

The Instant Calm Breath is a very short controlled breathing meditation, which is also one of the quickest and most effective ways to release tension and any uncomfortable emotion. I teach it to all my music students because it quickly frees your mind and body from the effects of nervousness. At the other end of the scale are horribly debilitating disorders like panic attacks—anyone can use the Instant Calm Breath to free themselves from such painful and frightening emotions. Like all Spot Meditations (see Chapter 6) it can be done any where, any time without anyone knowing what you are doing and it only takes 20 seconds.

Inner sensations and energy centres (chakras)

Meditations in this category are a more active form of meditation designed to move your focus to the *inner sensations* of your body. When these have opened up, you can concentrate directly on this inner world.

As you explore your inner sensations, you find that every emotion and sensation you experience tends to have a focal point in your body. The word often used for these focal points of energy or sensation is *chakra*. It literally means "wheel", and it represents a hub of sensation that radiates out like spokes. The most useful translation for this is "energy centre".

Unlike the impression many people have of chakras or energy centres, there are not a fixed number with fixed colours associated with them. Nor do they have direct and fixed equivalents with the physical organs and glands of our bodies. You will have a better understanding of energy centres if you view them as fluxing waves of sensation, constantly changing and shifting according to your mood.

This understanding is expressed in everyday sayings we take for granted. We speak of a good *belly laugh*, of having a *gut feeling* for something, or we might experience something as *gut-wrenching*. When we are nervous we have *butterflies in the stomach*. We find certain people *warm-hearted* and others *cold-hearted*. We can experience someone or something as a *pain in the neck*, and when we experience a strong emotion we say that our *throat feels choked up*. We can feel *clear*, *heavy* or *light-headed*.

Many people, as they open to deeper states of meditation, begin to see colours moving and swirling. They are beginning to open to their inner experience and will find that these colours are associated with moods and emotions. With practice, they can pinpoint the focal point in their bodies for these colours. Others will feel these sensations directly, rather than seeing images. So it's best to explore your own experience and discover for yourself how these energy centres operate.

Meditating on energy centres

There are two excellent meditations for beginning to understand the energy centres of your body—one is the Nourishing Breath meditation described at the end of this chapter; the other is the Bodyscan.

The Bodyscan meditation is done by starting at the top of the head and scanning through your body, becoming aware of all the sensations, whether pleasant, painful or neutral. It's helpful to do this meditation systematically in the six stages outlined later because it gives a clear focus and direction and opens up your awareness of the energy centres. You might be able to visualise the parts of your body as you scan through it and experience the sensations associated with them, or you might just feel the parts of your body without visualising them.

As you do this, you will notice your body relaxing, the muscles loosening and the fact that, as you allow your mind to accept the unpleasant feelings in your body, they move into the background and sometimes disappear altogether. This happens because your mind stops focusing on the thoughts and accompanying emotions you would normally have about pain or discomfort in your body, and the ideas about what you like about your body and what you don't like.

Instead, your mind is gently focusing on the sensations in your body, and you find yourself listening to what your body is *actually experiencing* rather than what you think it should or shouldn't be doing. It's quite a revelation when you do this, because you discover many areas in your body you normally don't notice. You also experience the relief and gentle bliss of your mind, body and emotions coming into balance and working in harmony.

Visualisation

Visualisation is another active form of meditation, which engages the imagination to create a specific feeling or state of mind. The Tibetan Tantric tradition is particularly rich in visualisations and many of these are aimed at getting to know, and learning how to access, all the different qualities of our minds.

Different ways to visualise

I have found that people either see clearly when meditating or they feel what they are imagining—and both are equally effective. So if you can *feel* what you are imagining, you are following a visualisation in the same way as someone who is actually seeing it.

Another question that often crops up in classes when people visualise, is *where* you actually see the image. Some people find they are right in their bodies, seeing the parts of their bodies as they scan or visualise. Others see the image in front of themselves—it's as though they are seated in a chair, watching the meditation in front of them. The key to all successful meditation is to accept what your body and mind are doing, even though it might not seem like the right or perfect thing to you.

You will find that visualisation begins to develop of its own accord as you practise and become used to it and your mind becomes ready to explore further.

Mind and Body Washing Meditation

The Mind and Body Washing Meditation is a visualisation that gives the mind and emotions a kind of "mental shower". It's a variation on the Bodyscan meditation, following the same steps, but includes a visual component as well. It involves becoming aware of the different parts of your body, and visualising or feeling them being washed through. It can be used to relax the muscles of your body, literally washing out all the unconscious tension we carry around. It can also be used for healing, which is powerfully effective when integrated with medical treatments.

Visual objects

Another way to meditate with the visual sense is to use a visual object. One way to do this is to create objects for formal meditation, for example, discs of colour, which are extremely effective for people who find it difficult to visualise colour. Or you might like to use a beautiful feather, flower, candle flame, crystal or semi-precious stone, which can bring you to a meditative state quickly and effectively. (These objects are outlined in detail in Chapter 22.)

The aim of meditating with a visual object is to use it as an anchor for your mind—giving it something to rest on so that it gradually becomes still. When your mind moves away, or gets caught in a thought, gently bring it back to the object. You might reach a point where you feel more comfortable with your eyes closed, and if so, allow this to happen—you may still hold an image of the object in your mind and see it quite clearly. As your meditation continues you might find yourself alternating naturally between opening and closing your eyes.

Mantra

Mantra is a Sanskrit word that comes from *mano* meaning mind, and *tra* meaning tool. Mantra, then, is a tool for training the mind. It also has the sense of something that protects the mind. Mantra is *meditating* on *sound* and this is one form of meditation flourishing in our culture. Music is the great mantra tradition of the West and I'm including in this all the different kinds of music we hear each day— popular, jazz, rock, classical, dance, rap, military and film music, and the world music of other cultures.

The word *music* is derived from the word *muse*. A muse in ancient Greek culture was a goddess who protected one of the arts or sciences. In English *muse* also means "to meditate on something". So music is a form of meditation.

When you are meditating on mantra, you are using a sound, or a series of sounds, or even a series of words, as a focus for your mind. Repeating a sound over and over holds your focus and allows you to let go of the constant undercurrent of thought that generally runs our lives. Mantras open your mind beyond its immediate concerns to views and ideas outside your self-interest, so that you feel yourself as an integral part of humanity and life.

Three categories of mantra

Mantras come in all shapes and sizes, from single syllables to very complex strings of words. In the Tibetan tantric tradition, all the visualisations have an accompanying mantra, and there are literally hundreds of different kinds. However, all mantras come in three distinct categories: **seed syllables, mixtures of visualisations and seed syllables,** and **contemplative**.

Seed syllables

These are mantras composed of sounds which have no meaning whatsoever. They are generally single syllables usually derived from Sanskrit, the ancient, classical language of India. Like music, they completely bypass our normal thought processes to resonate directly with feelings and emotions.

Many of these sounds can be found in English, such as **AH, MA, OH, HO, HA**. This is why they are called *seed syllables*, because they form the seeds of language. Although they have no meaning in themselves they can create certain associations in your mind and feelings in your body. For example, saying **AH** slowly generates a smooth feeling in the throat and falls into the body, whereas **HA**, because the H is at the beginning, is more emphatic as it involves the use of the diaphragm and rises up the body. **HO** has basically the same effect but seems to be lower in the body—we associate both **HA** and **HO** with laughter.

The simplest mantras can be just one syllable, like the famous **OM** (often spelt **AUM**) which is meant to encompass all vowels. Another simple mantra using three syllables is **OM AH HUM** (pronounced **OM AH HOONG**). **OM** has an opening effect in the head, **AH** is centred in the throat and falls into the body, and **HUM** resonates in the chest.

One effective way to feel the part of the body a seed syllable is focused in is to compare two different ones. If you take **HUM** and repeat it a few times slowly and then follow it immediately with the syllable **HRIH** (pronounced **HREE**) you will see what I mean. **HUM** creates a resonance in the chest that is very steady and solid, whereas **HRIH** is a very active sound which rises up through the body. An example of a longer mantra using all seed syllables is: **OM HRIH HA HA HUM HUM PHAT!**

Mixtures of visualisation and seed syllables

Most mantras fall into this category because they are usually composed of seed syllables and words that have meaning. The words are usually descriptive of what is being visualised in conjunction with the mantra. An example of this is the famous Tibetan mantra of compassion **OM MANI PADME HUM**. **OM** and **HUM** are seed syllables; many mantras begin with **OM**—focusing in the head to clear the mind and open it up, and ending with **HUM**—bringing the focus to the body and resting in the heart centre (in the middle of the chest).

MANI is pronounced **MARNEE**, and means "jewel". **PADME** is pronounced **PUDMAY** or **PAYMAY**, and means "lotus" or "flower". These words describe the visualisation of a red jewel seated within a large, open, white flower.

The jewel represents the mind, because it is crystal clear, can take on any colour and in its pure state, can reflect all the colours of the rainbow. In this case the jewel is red, which is the colour associated with love or compassion both in our culture and in Eastern cultures.

Throughout the meditation tradition, an open flower symbolises the body because like the body, and anything that grows, a flower begins its life as a seed and eventually grows and unfolds to become an open flower. This symbolises the fulfillment of its potential. It also has its roots in the earth because, like every living form, it is dependent on the earth for its survival.

The image of the jewel in the lotus represents the integration of mind and body. It demonstrates that our bodies have within them the open clarity of consciousness, so awareness, the ability to see, is *embodied*. Our minds can see and our bodies can act, and understanding their dependence on each other is the essence of love.

By using such a mantra, along with its accompanying visualisation, you train your mind to question and explore the experience of compassion, instead of taking for granted that you already know. Repeating the mantra provides a tool to recognise and access the quality of compassion at will. The visualisation, when repeated with the mantra during formal meditation sessions, engages the other senses, particularly visual and tactile, so that a very strong association is made with the mantra. This anchors a particular state of mind by touching the three ways we gather and process information—aural, visual and tactile.

After practising a mantra in this way, you build into your mind and body a set of associations that enable you to cultivate a particular state of mind and access it immediately.

Contemplative mantras

This category consists of mantras that are used to contemplate or reflect on ideas. We are very familiar with these kinds of mantras in advertising, where slogans become so well-known that almost everyone knows what company or brand is being referred to. One example of this is "Oh, what a feeling!"

Prayer comes under this category, as do affirmations. These mantras direct thought rather than attempting to go beyond thought. The Lord's Prayer is perhaps the most famous example of a contemplative mantra. Like all mantra, it uses sound—words—which are repeated the same way every time and focus the mind on particular ideas.

Affirmations—simple words or phrases you can use to focus your mind—are another conscious way of doing this. The best are those you create for yourself because you can tailor them to what you need in particular situations. For example, simple ones I have used in my own life are: **let go, love, be open, calm, peace, clear, be kind, alive**.

A traditional Buddhist contemplative mantra is **Araham Samma Sambuddho Bhagava**, which is a contemplation of the three stages of the inner path. The first stage is opening the mind and letting go of all concepts, symbolised by the word *Araham*. It is the initial stage of letting go of what is known. The second stage is the moment of illumination, when you directly experience the infinite luminosity of consciousness (*Samma Sambuddho*) and the third stage is one of unity, when this is integrated with your body and your life (*Bhagavan*).

An interesting version of contemplative mantra is the koan. This form is used in the Japanese Zen Buddhist tradition and, like all contemplative mantras, it provides an idea for the mind to focus on and contemplate, but paradoxically forces it to go beyond meaning. A famous example of a koan is "What is the sound of one hand clapping?" It appears to be a meaningless question; however, it creates such a paradox that it propels the mind beyond thought. There is an answer, but it has nothing to do with thought—it's a direct experience.

Movement

Movement has always been an integral part of the meditation tradition but most people don't know this, including many meditation teachers. Yoga, Tai Chi, Chi Gung and the martial arts all began as part of the meditation tradition. The Tibetan Buddhist tradition has a rich heritage of movement meditations called *Kum Nye* which we draw on extensively at The Lifeflow Meditation Centre.

Movement meditations are an invitation to become aware of, and feel, the dance of life both around you and within your own body. All forms of movement meditation begin by learning to balance the body, and then to maintain that balance no matter what position your body is in. This opens up the inner world of your sensations and as you explore these sensations through movement, you discover how to maintain a balanced state internally and then how to focus your mind at any point in your body. From here it is an easy step to meditate *directly* on the world of inner sensation.

While doing a movement meditation, concentrate on exploring all the sensations in your body—you will become acutely aware of the sensations in your arms, hands and fingers as you do the exercises outlined below. Notice everything, whether it feels pleasant, painful or neutral.

As you do the exercises and become more relaxed, you might begin to feel your body becoming heavier or lighter. You might also notice tingling sensations in your arms, fingers, or in your chest, or warmth in your body. You can sometimes begin to feel a huge space opening up around you. Your arms can feel as though they are moving by themselves—as though they become so light they are floating.

After a while, many people find they have become just as absorbed in movement meditation as in any other kind of meditation.

Contemplation

Meditations in this category are emotionally based and focus on ideas and images which inspire us and open us to a wider view of ourselves, beyond our usual boundaries. Opening up these boundaries is similar to opening the lungs and taking in a huge breath of fresh air—it refreshes and energises us.

We tend to live in a rather tight mental space and this not only separates us from the direct experience of our bodies, but also from feeling connected to others, to our community and to the environment in which we live. Contemplative meditations aim at rebuilding these connections so that we see ourselves not as isolated individuals in an alien universe, but as an integral part of life on this planet. Many contemplative meditations begin by accepting ourselves, our bodies and our lives, just as they are, which brings us back to earth.

A contemplative meditation can be developed from the state of balance we touch every time we meditate. This simple state, in which our bodies are still and relaxed, our emotions calm and our minds fairly peaceful, can be opened up to a deep sense of stillness. As you rest in this state you eventually come to see that you have completely let go of your identity and sense of self, and are resting in the core of your being, where your mind is open to everything equally, without judgment.

There are three kinds of contemplative meditations taught in the Lifeflow introductory course. The first is a meditation in which simple ideas are contemplated, to open to a feeling of being well and happy.

The second contemplative meditation we call Kindness and Acceptance. It begins by accepting yourself, just as you are—your body and your life—and then consciously generating feelings of kindness towards yourself. You might experience this as a sense of warmth or love and you extend this to all the parts of your body—those you like, those you don't like and those you usually take for granted.

This third contemplative meditation is a meditation on all-embracing kindness called The Ecology Meditation. This builds on the previous meditation by incorporating a visualisation which expands the feelings of kindness and accceptance to include others and then everything on which our bodies depend for their survival.

Insight

The seventh category of meditation is devoted to developing awareness or insight. The two meditations particularly well suited to developing awareness are Watching the breath and Bodyscan (both outlined earlier). These are ideal for "just watching"—you become aware of the movement of breath or sensations in the body without attempting to change them in any way, just seeing them as they are. In advanced practice you then move to just watching thoughts and emotions.

As you do this, you begin to notice the spaces between sensations, thoughts and emotions, and Insight meditation is the practice of focusing on and resting in that space, just watching everything coming and going (see also Chapter 15). Eventually your mind can open to the fundamental state of awareness—the foundation of the mind and the core of your being. You can experience your mind as completely still, clear and open and this enables you to see and understand the fundamental nature of your mind and consciousness—what the Buddhist tradition calls *Emptiness*.

There are four levels of directly experiencing how our minds and consciousness work, and the first level of insight is the moment of seeing your mind when it is empty of concepts—free from thoughts and emotions. This is the experience of the mind when it is completely still, open, aware of everything and vibrant and clear.

Instructions for meditations

Each time you prepare to meditate, follow the steps outlined in Chapter 2: rock gently to establish your balance point, run through the Bodycheck, and then open your mind to all the sounds around you. A short reminder is included in each category: *Rocking, Bodycheck, Sounds*.

Breathing meditations
Watching or feeling the breath

Rocking, Bodycheck, Sounds

Either half-close your eyes, or close them completely and bring your awareness to your nostrils. Watch or feel the breath moving in and out through your nostrils. If you have difficulty breathing through your nostrils, simply watch the breath moving in and out of your mouth. Feel the slightly cooler in-breath and the slightly warmer out-breath.

If you prefer, you can watch or feel the movement of your body as you breathe—the rise and fall of your chest or the movement of your abdomen.

Just follow your natural breathing. Notice if each breath is fast or slow, shallow or deep, short or long.

While doing this, bring your mind with the breath by saying silently to yourself, "breathing in" as you breathe in and "breathing out" as you breathe out.

You may notice thoughts or background sensations in the body—simply become aware of them, notice what they are, and then gently return to the breath.

When you are ready to finish the meditation, open your eyes slowly, and rest in the calm, balanced state of the meditation for a while before moving.

Counting each breath

You can also hold your attention on your breathing by counting each breath. Here are three options:

Rocking, Bodycheck, Sounds
1. Count on the out-breath from 1 to 10, then from 10 back to 1 again—breathe in, breathe out and count 1, then breathe in and out, 2, and so on. Repeat this for the duration of the session.
2. Silently say to yourself "breathing-in" as you breathe in and "breathing-out" as you breathe out. Then, count each out-breath from 1 to 10, then from 10 back to 1—"breathing-in, breathing-out, 1, breathing-in, breathing-out, 2" and so on.
3. Count from 1 to 10 and then back again from 10 to 1 by saying silently to yourself "and" on the in-breath, and counting the number on the out-breath—"And 1, and 2," and so on.

When you are ready to finish the meditation, open your eyes slowly, and rest in the calm, balanced state of the meditation for a while before moving.

Controlled breathing meditations
Instant Calm Breath

This meditation is in four steps:

1. Breathe out with a little sigh.
2. Take a deep breath in, just to where it is comfortable, feeling the movement of your abdomen.
3. Now hold your breath for a while—just as long as is comfortable for you.
4. Finally, and this is the important key, breathe out as slowly and smoothly as you are able.

Wave Breath

This meditation is particularly good for replenishing your energy and feeding yourself emotionally.

Rocking, Bodycheck, Sounds

Bring your awareness to your nose or mouth, feeling or watching the breath moving in and out through the nostrils. Notice the slightly cooler in-breath and the slightly warmer out-breath. Just follow your natural breathing.

Now become aware of the physical movement of your chest rising and falling with the breath.

Also notice the gentle movement of your abdomen as you breathe. Feel the physical movement of your whole torso breathing.

You may begin to feel the breath moving like a wave through your body. Imagine the movement of the breath soaking into and massaging your body.

When you are ready to finish, finish in the same way as for the other breathing meditations.

Nourishing Breath

This meditation is also good for replenishing your energy and feeding yourself emotionally—by expanding bliss and energy through your body.

Rocking, Bodycheck, Sounds

Bring your awareness to your nose or mouth, feeling or watching the breath moving in and out through the nostrils. Notice the slightly cooler in-breath and the slightly warmer out-breath. Just follow your natural breathing.

Now notice the physical movement of your chest rising and falling.

Also become aware of the gentle movement of your abdomen.

Feel your breath moving like a wave through your body.

The next time you breathe in, slightly slow down the in-breath. Follow it through to the centre of your chest.

When you breathe out, imagine the breath spreading through

your whole body—expanding through your chest, your neck and head, through your shoulders and arms, feeling it moving down through your belly and lower back, and down into your legs and feet. Then, if you like, you can imagine it leaving your body through the skin.

Continue this for three or four breaths.

Then follow the next in-breath through to the pit of your belly.

When you breathe out, follow the same process outlined in step 6.

Continue like this for three or four breaths, and see which is more comfortable for you—whether you prefer to follow the breath to the chest (the heart centre) or to the belly (the navel centre), and remain with that one. This will be the option to use each time you do this meditation.

Cultivate the feeling of drinking the breath into your body and allowing the breath to soak into your organs and muscles as you breathe out.

Finish the meditation by returning to the wave breath.

When you are ready to end the meditation, open your eyes slowly, and rest in the calm, balanced state of the meditation for a while before moving.

Energy centres
Nourishing Breath to explore energy centres

To use this meditation to explore energy centres, gradually move your focus from the breath itself to your heart or navel centre.

Become aware of the sensations generated in those centres and through your whole body.

Also, follow the in-breath from your nostrils up into your head, so you have the sense of breathing into your head.

This will allow you to come to know the three main energy centres in your body—head, heart and gut (navel).

Also notice any associated colours or images which arise.

Bodyscan

Rocking, Bodycheck, Sounds.

Start to become aware of the sensations at the top of your head, across the scalp, noticing any tingling, pressure or any other sensations.

Now bring your awareness to the forehead, to the eyes, down to the cheeks and jaw, and then the rest of your head. Notice all of the sensations—where it feels good, where there is pain or tension and where it is neutral so you are not particularly aware of anything. Also notice your breathing, so that you feel the breath moving in and out of your nostrils. Whether the sensations are pleasant or unpleasant, just let them be—just watching, noticing the subtle detail and any shifts or changes.

Take your awareness to your neck, your shoulders, your arms, hands and fingers.

Then notice all the sensations in your chest, feeling the movement of the ribs and chest as you breathe in and out. Then notice the sensations through the shoulders and upper back, feeling the muscles around the shoulder blades and along the length of your spine.

Move to the abdomen and lower back and notice all the sensations there.

Noticing all of the sensations—where it feels good, where there is pain or tension and where it is neutral so you are not particularly aware of anything. Whether the sensations are pleasant or unpleasant, just let them be, just watching the subtle detail and any shifts or changes.

Now take your awareness to your hips, your legs, your feet and toes.

After you have scanned your body, allow your mind to rest where it feels most comfortable—perhaps watching the breath at the chest or abdomen, or resting in a place which feels calm and where the sensation is neutral. You might find that you like to go through a systematic scan again, either from the top of your head or, having reached your feet, moving from there back up to your head.

Visualisation
Mind and Body Washing Meditation

Rocking, Bodycheck, Sounds

Imagine that it is a warm, sunny day, and that you are outside in a place where you can be alone and safe—somewhere that comes to mind immediately, either a memory from childhood or a place you know.

Gently allow the warmth of the air to soak into the muscles of your body, starting at the top of the head, across the scalp. Let it soak into your forehead, then move to the face and the whole head, then into your neck, throat, shoulders, arms and hands. Allow the warmth to gently soak into the muscles of your chest and upper back, your abdomen, hips, lower back and backside. Finally, allow the warmth to soak into the muscles of your legs and feet.

Then imagine a light, misty, warm shower of rain. The sun is still shining and the rain is filled with sunlight. Let it wash all over your body, feeling it flow over every part of your skin from the top of your head to your feet.

Then imagine it entering the top of your head and wash through the inside of your body. As it flows through your body, consciously take it to every part, as you wash hrough your whole body. See or feel it flowing into your scalp and the top of your head, your forehead and the whole of your face, then see or feel it flow into your neck and throat, shoulders, arms, hands and fingers and let it flow out the ends of your fingers.

Then allow it to flow into your chest and upper back, your abdomen and lower back and your hips, legs and feet and let it flow out the ends of your toes.

(If you are able, allow the detail of your body to come to mind—your bones, nervous and blood systems, your organs and muscles—as you let each part be washed through.)

Finish the meditation by allowing the whole visualisation to dissolve into light. This light enters and fills your body. Rest here for a moment feeling this soft light through your whole body.

When you are ready, gently open your eyes to come out of the meditation.

Some variations on this meditation:

Imagine yourself standing under a warm shower, filled with light.

Imagine yourself standing under a gentle, tropical waterfall in a beautiful part of nature.

Imagine a milky white liquid flowing from the centre of a cloud of light above your head.

Meditating on visual objects

Place the object about 1.5–2 metres in front of you so that when you look at it your eyes are looking down slightly. This helps both your eyes and mind to relax.

Rocking, Bodycheck, Sounds

Soften your eyes by allowing them to close and then open them slightly, so that they are half-open and your eye muscles feel relaxed. The area surrounding your meditation object will become slightly blurred when you do this.

Then allow your mind to rest on the object. This is quite subtle, and it's very different from looking at the object in a hard, concentrated way—just resting your gaze ensures you are not staring at the object, so that the muscles in your eyes and orehead can stay relaxed.

While you meditate, if you feel the need to blink or close your eyes, just do so, opening them again when you are ready. Notice if you can still see the object when your eyes are closed.

Example of a visual object meditation
One beautiful meditation using a visual object is to meditate on a piece of fruit, like an orange for example.

Place your hands in your lap with your left hand underneath your right hand. Hold the orange in your right hand so that you are looking comfortably down at it. Let your eyes soften, and then allow your mind to absorb the shape and colour of the orange.

As you go deeper into the meditation, imagine the past of the orange, allowing your mind to move through all the stages of the orange's birth and growth. And then let its future come to mind as you imagine where it is going and what will happen to it.

You can also do this meditation with the palm of your own hand:

Allow your mind to become absorbed in all the sense impressions your body is receiving about your hand. Notice its shape and the shapes of the fingers and thumb, the different colours and textures of the skin.

Then notice all the different lines on your hand. Allow your mind to become more deeply absorbed in the sense impressions of your hand. And then, as with the orange, open your mind to imagine the past and the future of your hand.

Mantra

The two mantras taught in Lifeflow's introductory course are **HAMSA** and **ARAHAM**.

Hamsa

Although it is not an exact translation, I give the meaning of "I am complete" for **HAMSA** because this gives a sense of its original meaning. This mantra creates a feeling of peace and calm.

To meditate on **HAMSA** begin by saying it out loud to yourself, pronouncing **HAM** as **HUM** and **SA** as **SAR**.

Say the **SAR** on your out-breath as a sigh that you can feel right through your body.

Then gradually let the mantra become silent (say it internally)

You will find you can then co-ordinate the **HUM** with the in-breath and the **SAR** with the out-breath.

Araham

The mantra **ARAHAM** embodies the sense of freedom—of being free from painful and conflicting emotions—so I give it the meaning "freedom". Most people find this mantra very energising.

To meditate on **ARAHAM**, pronounced **AH RA HUNG**, again begin by saying it out loud to yourself in three distinct syllables:
AH RA HUNG.
Then, when you are ready, let the mantra become silent so that you are saying it internally.

As you become used to these mantras you won't need to say them out loud, but can just let them rest in your mind so you can use them anywhere, anytime.

Movement meditations

These three short movement meditations are adapted from Tibetan Kum Nye exercises.

Raising and Lowering Shoulders

Put your hands on your thighs and then use your arms to raise your shoulders until they are as high as they will comfortably go.

Hold them there for a little while.

Then use your arms to lower your shoulders as slowly as you can.

When you think it is time to stop, keep going a little longer.

Flying

Stand well balanced with your feet shoulder-width apart, your back straight and your arms relaxed at your sides. Your eyes can be open or closed. If your eyes are open, gently soften the gaze by looking down a few metres in front of you.

Slowly lift your arms away from your sides in an arc around your body—feel the arms moving, feel the muscles working.

Take your arms above your head, letting your hands touch. When they do touch, have a little stretch.

Slowly take your arms back to your sides, following the same arc, keeping your awareness in the sensations of the movement.

When your arms are back at your sides, rest for a few moments, becoming aware of your breathing and of any sensations or feelings in your body any tingling, warmth or feeling of energy.

Repeat this movement two more times.

Swimming in Space

While standing, hold your hands straight out in front of you (at a right angle to your body), then slightly lift the left hand and lower the right.

Then lift the right and lower the left, letting them move a little further apart than before.

Keep repeating this movement, alternating lifting and lowering each hand while gradually letting the movement become larger and larger (so that your hands are moving further and further apart).

Keep repeating this until your arms are moving straight up and down.

Then gradually shorten each movement of your arms until your hands rest again in front of you.

Contemplation
Kindness meditation

Rocking, Bodycheck, Sounds

This is a short contemplation on kindness. As you run through the meditation, notice what thoughts, feelings or memories arise.

Simply repeat, either out loud or silently to yourself, the following four statements. *(These words are only a suggestion—you might find other words and ideas that you prefer.)*

May I be filled with kindness.

May I be well.

May I be peaceful and at ease.

May I be happy.

Now take any one of those ideas and stay with it, again noticing what images, feelings or memories arise out of it.

Acceptance and Kindness

Rocking, Bodycheck, Sounds.

Imagine in your heart centre a deep red rose bud. It opens to form a full rose: rich, deep red in colour. The petals have a velvety texture, and are covered in dew. See if you can feel the texture of the petals and smell their perfume. If you find that another kind of flower appears, or it is a different colour, just use this and stay with what you see or feel.

From this rose comes a soft, pale pink light that spreads into your head and neck, chest, shoulders, arms and hands, and then into your whole torso, hips, legs and feet. With this light come warm feelings of kindness, acceptance and love towards your whole body and your life. Let these feelings grow.

Become aware of all the effort your body makes to stay alive and stay well, its constant work even when you are asleep, That it has to eat and breathe, that it lives within limits, and that it shares this effort with everybody and everything that lives on this planet. Also bring to mind that your body is totally dependent on the earth for its life.

Bring your awareness to the parts of your body which are comfortable and which work well. Let the light, along with the feelings of kindness and warm love, soak deeply into them.

Now notice those parts of your body which are uncomfortable, which may cause tension and pain. For the moment, allow yourself to accept them just as they are, as an integral part of your body. Extend the light to these areas and allow it to soak in deeply bringing feelings of acceptance, kindness and love.

Now bring your awareness to those parts of your body which you normally don't notice and take for granted. Again, bring the light to these areas, allowing it to soak in deeply. With it come feelings of acceptance, kindness and warm love.

Open to the realisation that all these areas form an integral part of your body, sharing equally in the effort it makes to stay alive and healthy.

See and feel the light soaking deeply into your whole body along with the feelings of acceptance, warmth, kindness and a deep sense of peacefulness.

Let the rose at your heart centre dissolve into the light in your body and rest with these feelings through your whole body. Then, letting go of the light, gently come out of the meditation.

The Ecology Meditation—All-embracing Kindness

Rocking, Bodycheck, Sounds

Imagine in your heart centre a deep red rose bud. It opens to form a full rose: rich, deep red in colour. The petals have a velvety texture, and are covered in dew. See if you can feel the texture of the petals and smell their perfume. If you find that another kind of flower appears, or it is a different colour, just use this and stay with what you see or feel.

From this rose comes a soft, pale pink light that spreads into your head and neck, chest, shoulders, arms and hands, and then into your whole torso, hips, legs and feet. With this light come warm feelings of kindness, acceptance and love towards your whole body and your life. Let these feelings grow.

Expand the light to form a sphere of light around you, so that you are held and supported by this warm feeling of love, kindness and acceptance. (If you wish, you can remain here.)

You can then expand the light in stages so that it fills the room you are in, then the building, the city and the country, embracing everybody who lives there with the same warmth and kindness. Embrace all the animals and birds, the trees and plants, all the creatures that live in the soil, sea and air. Bring to mind the understanding that all these different beings live within the same limitations as your own body and experience the same struggle to live.

As you complete each stage, rest there for a while embracing all the different forms of life in this light and feeling of kindness and understanding.

Now expand the light to embrace the whole earth—all the different continents, oceans, people of different races, creeds and colours, and all the animals, trees, plants and creatures who live in the soil, air and sea. Rest here for a while, understanding that everybody and every form of life are interconnected and dependent on the earth for their survival.

Then gradually bring the light back in stages to your own body. Rest for a while either seeing or feeling this light filling your whole body.

Then gently open your eyes and come out of the meditation.

Insight Meditation
Following a natural movement

This is a meditation you can do at any time.

Simply become aware of any movement you are making—such as lifting a cup of coffee to drink, opening a door, walking along a corridor, picking up a pen, and so on.

Become aware of the moment you begin the movement and then follow it right through to its completion.

For example, follow the movement of lifting the cup of coffee, placing it to your lips, tasting and drinking the coffee, and putting the cup back on the table.

The next chapter explores what happens as you move into the deeper stages of meditation.

Chapter 5: The deepening stages of meditation

The ability to be calm and clear is the foundation of a useful and happy life.

Every time you settle down to meditate, your mind goes through three stages: noticing how busy your mind is; seeing the space between thoughts and finally, the thoughts stopping altogether. As you become increasingly familiar with this, you will notice that it also happens every time you begin to concentrate. This chapter discusses the deepening stages of meditation and describes how to recognise an absorbed state.

Stage 1—Noticing the busyness

The first thing you notice as you begin to meditate is how active your mind is. You become acutely aware of how much traffic goes through it; how busy your thoughts are and how much they feed off each other. At this point people often become discouraged and think their meditation is not working or is getting worse. Actually it's getting better! It's a clear sign that you have entered a meditative state, calmed down, and begun to concentrate.

You are no longer caught in your normal thought processes. As you enter this first stage, becoming balanced and calm, you become aware of the undercurrent of thought which is always in the mind. You become aware of your thoughts as objects separate from yourself for the first time, and this is why it can be so alarming. You can watch them, without having to do anything about them, so you can actually see your thoughts instead of being driven by them. (This is a very useful state for everyday life, because you become aware of what you are thinking and what is happening.)

As you rest with this awareness you progress to the next stage, where it seems as though your thoughts are slowing down.

Stage 2—Seeing the spaces between thoughts

At this second deepening stage of meditation, there aren't so many thoughts, there is plenty of space between them, and you can see them coming and going. You will feel much calmer, and from this point meditation flows effortlessly. You experience a sense of peace through your whole body.

At this point you have entered an absorbed state; your mind becomes totally absorbed in the meditation object. These absorbed states are often called *transpersonal states, alternate states of consciousness* or *trance states*. They are often made to sound strange, and in Buddhism can be idealised so that they seem to be unattainable or at least rare.

However, we experience these states quite naturally during our everyday lives. They occur when we are very interested in something, when something absorbs our mind completely and when we "switch off" from what is happening around us. We may be watching a film, reading a book, playing sport, listening to music, working, walking, swimming or surfing and experience those magic times when we "zone out" and completely lose track of time.

We become totally engaged in what we are doing, and it's as though we are no longer there. We may have the sense that what we are doing is *doing itself*, or that we have become an integral part of the landscape. Things become brighter and clearer. Our mind is alert and lucid and completely free from any emotional disturbance.

In this state we talk about being *absorbed*. The word *absorb* comes originally from the Latin word *absorbere* which means "to suck in". So being in an absorbed state is like sucking something into the mind, drinking it in. Meditation is exactly like that: opening the senses and drinking everything in, so we are right there with what is happening.

I've found that every student and client can remember a time in childhood when they experienced this. Unfortunately it is hardly ever encouraged in our culture—children are told off for "daydreaming"— so many of us have learned to ignore this state or not take it seriously. And yet in this state, the human mind is at its most productive, creative and happy. An absorbed state is the foundation of meditation, because the ability to be calm and clear is the foundation of a useful and happy life.

Stage 3—The thoughts stop

As you enter an absorbed state of meditation you feel your mind and emotions becoming increasingly still. As the mind becomes calmer and more concentrated it becomes balanced, and it does this by resting on the meditation object instead of rushing from one object to another. The more focused our minds are, the more relaxed and calm we become. Eventually it reaches a point where it is no longer thinking about the object—or anything else—but is *resting totally in the sense experience*. This is a state of deep peace. For a moment or two, the thinking stops.

Waves in the sea

I have previously compared thoughts and emotions with waves in the sea. So let's look at the three deepening stages of meditation again, using this comparison.

Stage 1—Seeing the waves and currents

Usually we don't take much notice of our thoughts and emotions, so we go wherever they propel us—they form the undercurrent driving our lives. This is exactly like floating in the sea, without noticing where the currents are going, and ignoring the waves—until a big one comes along, throws us around and eventually breaks, taking us with it.

Becoming aware of these waves while they are still ordinary, everyday waves is the first deepening stage of meditation. We notice for the first time that they are present most of the time—just coming and going, pushing us around with them.

This moment of seeing means we have become calm enough or, in other words, the sea has settled down enough, for us to notice the waves—the calm provides a clear comparison.

Stage 2—Coming into harbour

When the sea becomes fairly still, we notice every wave as it comes and goes. We can see a wave before it reaches us, we can ride over it without any trouble, and we can see it leaving. The sea is so still that there are quite long stretches between waves. The feeling in meditation at this stage is rather like coming into a protected harbor where the sea is tranquil.

Stage 3—Finding the beach

Finding the beach is a profound experience of discovering there is somewhere free from waves, where it is possible to stay perfectly still, completely relaxed and deeply peaceful.

Knowing there is a beach makes all the difference to our attitude to the sea. Once we know there is somewhere free from the pushes and pulls of currents and waves, we know that when the going gets a bit rough we can get out and wait for the waves to settle down again.

Later, if we want to ride waves and feel the thrill of jumping into surf, we have the resources to do it because we know how to get out. And if we want to study the sea beforehand, we have a place to observe its patterns. Naturally, this is the same for our thoughts and emotions. They move through our minds like waves on the sea, and when you enter stage 3, you discover that there is a beach—a place completely free from them.

Recognising the deepening stages of meditation

Each time you meditate you will naturally move up and down these stages, often not noticing that you have become completely still until you return to stage 1. So the way to recognise the deepening stages of meditation is to notice when you come out of them. Hold yourself in that space for a little while to get a feeling for where you have been.

By paying attention to these stages in meditation, you will gradually be able to recognise what is happening as you meditate and gain more confidence and skill in calming your mind, so that it is not dominated by thinking. Use the quick summary below to help recognise the stages.

Summary of the three deepening stages of meditation:

1. You notice how busy your mind is as you see thoughts rushing around. You are watching your thoughts instead of being driven by them—so you *disengage* from them.

2. Your thoughts slow down so that you can see them coming and going. You become aware of spaces between the thoughts.

3. Your mind and emotions become so balanced that your thinking pauses for a while.

The qualities of an absorbed state

As you enter the second deepening stage of meditation and come to know its qualities you will be able to recognise an absorbed state and achieve it at will. There are five qualities which characterise an absorbed state.

1. Your thinking becomes clear and effective and stays with whatever you are focusing on, without being easily distracted.
2. Your emotions are calm and you are naturally interested in what is happening and feel a sense of pleasure, which can become joyful or even ecstatic.
3. Your body becomes very relaxed, becoming increasingly still until it happily stays completely still—there is no need to move. Your body may feel heavier, or in some cases, lighter, and a sense of deep peace and physical bliss will arise.
4. Your mind is focused with "one-pointed" concentration, which means it does not wander off. If it does, it's very easy to bring it back again because it doesn't wander off too far.
5. You are in a state of balance: physically, emotionally and mentally. Your meditation flows easily.

One of the ultimate aims of meditation is to be able to contact this absorbed state in everyday life, where life flows smoothly as you travel with it, connected with your body, your senses and the life around you.

As you develop your practice you might like to explore further all the different meditative states it is possible to experience. (See Chapter 12 for a detailed explanation of the different levels of absorption.)

The next chapter explores how you can touch the deep stillness of the meditative state to find your balance whenever you choose, using Spot Meditations.

Chapter 6: Spot Meditations

Spot Meditations are the wedge that allows you to find a moment to consciously relax and calm your mind.

Every time you meditate, even if you only *lightly* touch the meditative state, it creates enough space for your mind and body to return to their natural state of balance. In this calm state your energies are refreshed and your mind can watch and see clearly what is happening.

Spot Meditations are a way to very quickly gain this balance anywhere, any time, no matter what is happening. They can be done in twenty seconds or less and allow you to apply the skills you have learned in meditation to the thick of everyday life—right in the heat of the moment. They are ideal for creating some space and peace during the day and even for changing ingrained habits.

No matter how busy they are, we find that our students use Spot Meditations, because even if they can't find time to meditate formally, they find it easy to incorporate one or two Spot Meditations a few times each day. At home and at work, at meetings, between appointments, between clients, while having tea or coffee, while parked in the car, while at stop lights, on the bus or train, these little meditations can have a lasting effect on the quality of your day.

This is invaluable when you have a busy schedule and find it difficult to make clear divisions between tasks, home and work, day and night, which can become such a blur that life seems relentlessly the same. Using Spot Meditations to make these divisions will greatly improve the wellbeing of your mind and body.

A repertoire of Spot Meditations

Here are a range of very useful, tried and tested Spot Meditations. Some use breathing and others incorporate breathing and movement, use visualisation, mantra or sound or focus on the sensations of your body. Choose one or two of your favourites and make them a regular event in your daily life so you can quickly find your balance whenever you need to.

Meditating on Sound

This meditation, which we use at the beginning of every formal meditation, can be used on its own as a Spot Meditation when you are outside in a garden, walking in a park, on the beach or any other natural environment.

Open your mind to all the sounds around you.

Listen out as far as you can, listening to all the sounds just as sound. Allow every sound into your awareness.

You might hear sounds in your own body; perhaps the sound of your heart beating or the sound of the breath moving in and out of your body; if so, open up to them as well.

You may also feel your body resonating with the sounds around you. Let the feelings of the sound go through your whole body.

Allow your awareness to rest in the sensation of sound.

Let yourself be held by the sensation of sound—you might even have a sensation of floating in sound.

When you are ready to finish, just come back to feeling the contact of your body with the ground, chair or wherever you are.

Rocking Side to Side

Rocking also forms an integral part of each formal meditation in this book. It is a very simple way to gain your physical balance point and deepen the feeling of balance through your body and mind, so it can also be used as a Spot Meditation.

While sitting, gently rock your torso from side to side. Feel the movement along the length of your spine and focus on the physical sensations in your body.

As you rock from side to side, gradually allow the movement to get smaller and smaller.

Like a pendulum coming to rest, your body will naturally find its own balance point, so allow your body to become still of its own accord. When it does become still, open your mind to this feeling, where your torso is resting at the mid-way point between your hips.

Now gently rock your head and neck from side to side, again allowing this movement to get smaller and smaller until your head gradually comes to rest at the mid-way point between your shoulders.

Feel how your spine is aligned through your neck, chest and abdomen as it rests at the point mid-way between your hips. Notice the feeling of balance through your whole body.

Contact Points

This Spot Meditation can be used when you first get into a car or at stoplights; when you are sitting on a bus, train or tram; at work, when you are at meetings or just sitting at a desk. You can do it with your eyes open. You can also adapt it for lying down in bed or any other time you are lying on your back.

These instructions are for sitting in a chair.

Begin by becoming aware of the position of your body. Feel the contact of your feet on the floor, the back of your thighs on the chair, your backside on the chair, your back on the backrest, and the position of your arms and hands—feeling the contact on your thighs, lap or arm rests of the chair.

Now, move your awareness to your left foot, and allow a feeling of it sinking into the floor.

Now let your right foot sink into the floor.

Allow the back of your left thigh to sink into the chair, and the back of your right thigh to sink into the chair.

Let your backside also sink into the chair.

Feel your back on the backrest and let yourself have the feeling of slightly falling back into the chair.

Finally, let your arms and hands rest into your thighs or lap, feeling the weight of your hands resting on your legs, or on the arm rests of the chair.

Rest here for a while, as long as you wish.

Raising and Lowering Shoulders

This Spot Meditation is a shorter version of a movement meditation, where you raise your shoulders until they are almost tense, then lower them slowly and deliberately.

Place your hands on the top of your thighs.

Raise your shoulders by pushing your hands against your thighs, until both of your shoulders are lifted as high as possible.

When you think your shoulders are as high as they can be, relax your body, and you may find your shoulders can move up a little more.

Hold this posture for a few moments—breathing naturally.

Now, using your arms, very slowly begin to lower your shoulders until they are back to the position where you started the exercise. The key to this Spot Meditation is bringing the shoulders down slowly, feeling the sensations all the way.

Feel the tension releasing little by little. When you think your shoulders are down, see if you can let them go a little further still.

Now rest here for a few moments, becoming aware of your breathing and of any sensations or feelings in your body; any tingling, warmth or feeling of energy, noticing the sensations in your shoulders, neck or around your back.

Simple Hand Massage

This is a very useful way to make contact with your body without anybody noticing.

Place your left thumb on the thick, fleshy part between the thumb and forefinger of your right hand.

At the same time place the forefinger of your left hand underneath this part and use the thumb and forefinger to massage this part of your right hand.

Then, in the same way, massage your left hand using the thumb and forefinger of your right hand.

Standing

While you are standing waiting for a bus or friend is an excellent time to do this Spot Meditation. If you have the kind of job that requires you to be on your feet a lot, such as nursing or working in a store, you don't have to go away to meditate, you can take ten to twenty seconds while you are standing.

As you are standing, bend your knees slightly and become aware of the physical feeling of your body as you do this. This lowers your centre of gravity and literally grounds you while allowing your body to relax a little.

This works particularly well when combined with the Simple Hand Massage.

Sigh!

This Spot Meditation uses a natural reflex of the body.

Take a deep breath in.

Then breathe out with a long, slow sigh.

As you sigh, feel it going right through your body. You might even be able to feel the effect right through to your hands and feet.

Instant Calm Breath

In this Spot Meditation you use your breathing in a controlled way to quickly calm your emotions and restore a state of balance. It is particularly useful for those people who like meditating on the breath.

The Instant Calm Breath is done with your eyes open and no-one will notice you doing it. This meditation is in four steps:

1. Breathe out with a little sigh.

2. Take a deep breath in, just to where it is comfortable, feeling the movement of your abdomen.

3. Now hold your breath for a while—just as long as is comfortable for you.

4. Finally, and this is the important key, breathe out as slowly and smoothly as you are able.

Concentration

This is a variation on the Instant Calm Breath which is particularly useful when you need to hold your focus very still. It can help you establish and sustain a totally focused state of concentration, so is invaluable for study, exams, sport and other times you need to be particularly sharp.

For sharpening your concentration, follow steps 1 to 3 of the Instant Calm Breath then:

Let your breath out smoothly and slowly, and as you do this, imagine your breath coming out through the middle of the forehead.

You can either visualise the breath as a stream of light, or feel it.

Bodyline

This Spot Meditation is particularly useful for those who can visualise easily. It's a very quick way to balance your mind and emotions by bringing your focus back to your body. It can create a feeling of being alert and centred, and is very useful for sustaining your concentration at work or while playing sport.

You can leave your eyes open and no-one will notice that you are meditating.

Imagine or visualise a line, or column of light, through the centre of your body. You can imagine it as quite thin and sitting just in front of your spine.

Follow it from the top of your head, through your neck, into your chest and down to the pit of the abdomen.

You may either see or feel this, and you will be able to do it very quickly.

Smiling Breath

This Spot Meditation uses a natural reflex of your body and your breathing to quickly calm your emotions and create a feeling of joy. It can be done whenever you have some time to yourself.

Close your eyes.

Now, deliberately put a smile on your face.

Count the next three breaths, in and out. "Breathing in—breathing out, one; breathing in—breathing out, two; breathing in—breathing out, three".

Let your breathing return to normal.

Open your eyes and notice how you feel. You may find that your emotions have settled, or notice a gentle feeling of joy in your body.

HAMSA (pronounced HUM SAR)

Repeat the mantra silently to yourself, using HUM on the in-breath and SAR on the out-breath.

You can let the SAR be like a sigh, feeling it move down through your body.

Simple Shoulder Stretch

Here is a way to quickly release the tension that can build up in your neck and shoulders. It can be used at work to refresh and balance yourself regularly during the day. You can do it sitting or standing.

Breathe in and pull your shoulders up tightly, deliberately tensing the shoulder muscles.

Then take your shoulders back and hold them there for a little while.

Now, while allowing your mind to focus on the physical sensations in your body, slowly let your shoulders down, breathing out with a sigh as they relax.

Rest here for a moment, noticing the feeling of relaxation through your shoulders, and maybe through your neck. You might feel a sense of relaxation through your whole body.

Simple Neck Massage

This Spot Meditation is based on a natural movement we often do through the day—reaching up to feel or massage the neck. What makes it a Spot Meditation is that you rest your mind on the actual sensations for a few seconds.

Using one hand, grip the back of your neck with the heel of the palm and the fingers of your hand.

Explore the sensations in your palm and fingers ... then gently massage into the neck muscles.

Work the fingers into the neck muscles, gently softening any areas that feel tight or overworked.

Let your hand rest back by your side.

Then, if you wish, repeat the exercise, using the other hand.

When you have finished massaging your neck, let your hands and arms relax and spend a few moments noticing the sensations through your neck. You might feel a sense of warmth, tingling, or energy. You may notice a sense of softening through the neck, and through the upper shoulders or back of the head.

This meditation is very effective for people who suffer from headaches and migraines, because it helps prevent the chronic build-up of tension in the neck muscles.

The next chapter explores how you can apply the moment of meditative space gained from a Spot Meditation to situations in your everyday life. It's called the **Three C Technique**.

Chapter 7: The Three C Technique

Bringing awareness to something, just watching it without doing anything about it, allows you to actually see what you are doing and accept it.

An integral part of Lifeflow meditation is the **Three C Technique**. This practical technique can be used in any situation in which you are beginning to get caught in an emotional habit pattern. It can be done quickly in the heat of the moment, to defuse a difficult situation, or be practised at greater length in formal meditation or on retreat. It can also be used to check the mental and emotional "weather" before making decisions or doing something demanding (see Chapter 14).

There are three steps: **Catch the moment, Clear the space and Change the habit**.

Catch the moment

This first step is a moment of acceptance—*of opening up to what is happening and to what you are doing.* It's a moment of simply admitting: "I'm angry, I feel sad, I'm afraid, I'm out to get this at all costs, I'm lost, I feel stressed or I don't understand what's happening ..."

Catching the moment is easier than it seems because often we are aware when we are about to go down a familiar emotional road. It's just that we usually don't have the knowledge or resources to do anything about it, so the habit takes over. The old song, "Falling in love again... I can't help it" sums this up beautifully. You might have started to say something you know you will regret later, but can't stop yourself, or you might experience an emotion you know has the potential to overwhelm you, or you might have started to react physically to something, thinking "To hell with the consequences", even though you know the outcome will be disastrous.

Most of the time we feel there is nothing we can do so we soldier on and do the same old thing, or we give up. However, there is something we can do and this is where the discipline of meditation really comes into its own.

The second step in the **Three C Technique** is to:

Clear the space

Clearing the space is what meditation is for, *par excellence*. It's a tool for balancing yourself so that you have space to watch and be aware, to stay still instead of feeling you have to do something immediately and to see what is happening. (Immediately reacting is sometimes appropriate, but more often this moment of balance and stillness is far more effective than your habitual reaction.)

All this takes is a quick Spot Meditation. Any familiar one will do, so you can find your balance—because if you are headed in a habitual direction you can be fairly sure you are completely off-balance. Clearing some space brings back the broader context and frees your mind from tunnel-vision. It disengages your emotions from the situation for a moment, so you are free to move in another direction or not at all if you so decide.

The final step in the process is to:

Change the habit

Changing the habit will happen almost automatically, because when you clear some space through meditating, you will be able to see through and around the situation you are in, and will nearly always find an alternative to your habitual way of reacting.

One student was so excited about her first experience of applying this technique she had to share it with the other students in the course. She owned a shop and one morning, while the shop was full and she was extremely busy, a woman came into the shop demanding attention, obviously very angry about something. This was a real test because, as our student freely admitted, she herself was very feisty and would normally have ended up in an argument. She was fully in the spotlight but quickly did her Spot Meditation and instead of engaging as she normally would have, she became very calm. For the first time in her life she did not panic or get angry.

She described it as her mind suddenly letting go and becoming emotionally detached from what was happening, so she could stay still and watch. Each time the woman paused for breath in her litany of complaints, she simply reassured her that she was there to help. Eventually the woman stopped and became quiet, turned around and quietly left the shop. There was no confrontation or fight. The other customers spontaneously burst into applause and as the student said, "I lost one customer but gained everyone else in the shop".

Combining the two types of concentration

The **Three C Technique** combines both types of concentration: opening and focusing.

Opening

The first step of **Catching the moment** is simply becoming aware of what you are actually doing instead of what you *think* you're doing, or *hope* you're doing. It's a moment of awareness where you allow your mind to *open* to the periphery and let go of the ideas you are focused on. This awareness allows you to catch the emotion or thought that is driving you.

You might pick up an uncomfortable sensation or emotion, or see the reaction of the person you are with. You might also feel that you are pushing hard to keep going where you want to go, or perhaps feel you are spinning out of control.

Bringing awareness to something, just watching it without doing anything about it, allows you to actually *see* what you are doing and accept it.

Focusing

A quick Spot Meditation automatically **Clears the space**. It does this by *focusing* your mind on your senses, which brings your mind and emotions to a point of balance. You literally come to your senses. This clears the mind of thoughts and emotions inherent in your habitual reaction to the situation, and gives you room to just watch what is happening—both within and outside of yourself.

This is a crucial step, and often the last thing you would ever think of doing. When we are caught in a habitual reaction and become aware of it, we want to do something about it, and this is where we dig ourselves in deeper. Instead, you balance yourself, letting your mind and emotions become as still and calm as possible under the circumstances.

Seeing what is happening

From this position of balance it is possible to **Change the habit**. Instead of the mind being focused on the habit it has calmed and become clearer. It is now resting in what is *actually* happening and what you are *actually* feeling, instead of being focused on the *idea* of what is happening and the emotion this creates. Your body is brought into awareness and your mind is anchored in your senses—it is now possible to make a clear decision about what to do, or what not to do.

Have you ever noticed that when you decide to change a habit, invariably you are focused on the habit itself? For example, if you decide to give up chocolate or smoking, your mind becomes obsessed with chocolate or smoking. A resolution is made, and you tend to think that you have done the work—the habit should change. The problem is that because your mind is still thinking about the habit, you will inevitably continue down the same path, as your mind hasn't been given the space to conceive an alternative.

In institutions and workplaces where a decision is made to change something, people often focus on the idea of what they want to happen. A paper is written to detail all the changes, speeches are given, and then nothing happens on the ground. Things go on as they were, because the emotions of the people involved and the habits that have been built up in the organisation are not taken into account. This is like moving deck chairs around on *The Titanic* hoping that somehow it will change the direction of the ship. For that you have to go to the engine room, and leave the deck. Similarly, you need to get to the space in your mind, which clears your mind of its normal ways of thinking about what it is you want to change. In this space you will find the alternative.

Your mind needs space to see something differently—it can then become detached from its normal way of seeing, and open to a different perspective. It's exactly like going into the bush to watch birds or animals in the wild. If you crash around looking for them they will keep out of your way. If you stay still, with your mind and senses wide open, they will gradually reveal themselves.

Stepping back and becoming free from habits

Becoming free from habits is one of the unique advantages meditation offers. Through meditation you can open up space between yourself, the habit and the situation you are in. You can then see beyond the fixed object in view to the context in which the object or situation is operating, and therefore see alternatives. Just doing this changes the habit, *because opening up this moment of space is itself the change*. It can be surprising how different a situation looks when this happens; often you can see an alternative that would never normally occur to you.

Instead of someone being a threat, you might suddenly see their pain. Instead of feeling you are at a dead end you might discover an alternative route around the situation, which would normally be impossible to imagine. You might see aspects of another person for the first time and find that this opens up a new way to communicate. Or you might see there is no way forward and instead of getting into a fight, remain silent or quietly turn around and leave. Any of these options, and more, is possible once you Clear the space to let go of your normal habitual reaction.

Many students and clients completely change relationships at home and work, and free themselves from anxiety, panic attacks, depression, stress or worry by giving themselves space to change their habitual reactions. With the **Three C Technique** they can Catch the moment the habit is about to kick in or, in other words, they are able to see the wave coming before it actually catches them. Then, by using a Spot Meditation that will instantly balance their mind and emotions and create a moment of calm and space, they are freed from going down their habitual path. *The habit has changed.*

When you begin to use this technique, you often don't notice what is happening until you are well into your usual reaction. It doesn't matter *when* you Catch the moment—it only matters that you eventually do. As soon as you Catch the moment, you will be able to do your Spot Meditation and so Clear the space.

As you become more skilled, you will Catch the moment sooner, until eventually you will see the habit coming, before it has taken hold.

The next chapter shows you how to deal with the emotion you catch using the **Three C Technique**—how to discharge it effectively or just stay still, learn how it works and how to transform it.

Chapter 8: Letting go of emotions

We are trained not to act on strong emotions so we feel a certain amount of guilt about having them. Nice people simply don't have these kinds of feelings. So we have to give up being nice and remember that our bodies are not nice—they are real!

Even after successfully applying the **Three C Technique** in an emotionally-charged situation, the emotion might still be there. This technique doesn't guarantee that the emotion will go away—it provides the space not to get caught in it or be forced to act on it.

If you are still seething with anger, for example, after the situation has passed, it is possible to discharge the emotion safely. You have become aware of the emotion, balanced yourself, and been spared the consequences of being driven by it. Therefore, the emotion is contained within your own mind and body rather than exploding into the environment around you. Now it is possible to deal with it.

There are two ways to do this: discharge it, which is an excellent short-term solution, or use meditation to stay still with the emotion, understand how it works, and use techniques to transform it.

Discharging an emotion

Anger is a useful emotion to examine because it is highly charged with energy and potentially explosive. We usually learn to deal with strong emotions like anger by attempting to resist them, so it's not surprising we become stuck.

Instead of finding possible reasons for the anger, fear, lust, hatred, anxiety, conflict, agitation, jealousy or other strong and painful emotion we feel (whether justifiable or not) the exercise for discharging emotion focuses on its direct effect on the body.

We are usually unaware of the effect emotions have on our bodies, but meditation provides the balance and calm to become aware of these effects. Any time we experience an emotion it means our minds are stuck in a particular thought pattern and the muscles of our bodies have become tense. Anger makes your body tight and constricted, with the muscles around the abdomen particularly tense.

In tantric terms, when we experience a painful emotion like anger, our energies have literally become blocked and can't flow freely, so finding a way to allow the body to complete the movement (release the energy) will discharge the emotion. Instinctively we've all done this in the past by getting the body moving; chopping wood was one old-fashioned and extremely effective way.

Years ago at The Lifeflow Meditation Centre we kept a woodpile, axe and old dinner plates for the purpose of discharging strong and painful emotions. One woman who suffered from frustration and anger was almost speechless when I gave her a plate and suggested she hurl it at the ground. It took a lot of encouragement but eventually she did it. Afterwards her body was visibly shaking as it released years of in-built tension. She then burst out laughing.

Failing spare dinner plates, there is another way to safely and effectively discharge strong emotion; it's called **The Pow Technique**.

The POW Technique

This exercise is drawn from the tantric tradition, but is adapted and simplified.

Instructions for POW!

Stand with the feet about shoulder-width apart and the knees very slightly bent. This is the martial arts stance, which provides optimum balance when you are standing.

Then make a fist with your dominant hand.

Bend the knees further so that you move into a crouch, bending slightly forward and twisting towards your dominant side. You will notice that this brings your body into a position where the muscles of the abdomen are deliberately tightened and brought into focus.

Now punch across your body, in front of your abdomen, with a sharp uppercut while shouting **POW!**

Repeat this twice more.

We teach this exercise in our introductory course and without exception, everyone bursts out laughing. One student taught it to her children and she told me they loved it so much they used it frequently. A teenage girl suffering trauma from an attack looked at me very strangely as I showed her this exercise, but when she did it her enthusiasm was unbounded. She loved the uppercut and shouting

POW! and could feel the release of tension and fear in her body.

What everyone notices when they are asked to check how they feel, is that the emotion has gone. Laughter and yawning are the signs of tense muscles in the abdomen letting go. The diaphragm is then freed up and the breathing deepens, drawing fresh air deeply into the lungs and expelling the stale air.

One student had been in a life-threatening situation where a homemade bomb was thrown at her. She lived with it for years and despite counseling could not let go of the fear. It took her some time and encouragement to even attempt this exercise. However, after doing it, she immediately began sobbing and had to sit down as her body began shaking. Then she looked at me utterly astounded as she said: "My throat is opening up! Oh, my chest is opening up!" And then she started yawning deeply. At the end of the session she said, "I can't believe it was that quick and simple!"

A variation for more resistant emotions

If an emotion like anger has become a habitual problem, there is another exercise, similar but not so portable.

> Kneel down by the side of a bed.
>
> Make fists with both hands and raise both arms while bending backwards slightly so that the hands are behind the head.
>
> Then bring the fists down onto the bed in a chopping motion while shouting **POW!**
>
> Again this releases the tension in the abdomen.
>
> Repeat this a few times.

The two POW! exercises move the blocked energy of strong emotion up through your body so it can be released. The first does it by punching your fist in an uppercut while your body moves from a crouch upwards. The second exercise does it by lifting your arms from behind your back, up and over your head. Yelling POW! focuses your energy in the belly and forces the muscles to release. It also opens your throat and causes you to breathe right down into the abdomen, releasing the tension there.

The other technique for dealing with an emotion in the longer term is to stay still and watch it, learn how it works and how to transform it.

Staying still

The great discovery of the meditation tradition is that keeping your body still will cause any emotion or state of mind, no matter how disturbed, to become calm and settled. This is so simple that you might wonder why there's an entire tradition built around it. Firstly, even though the principle is so simple, it's not easy to do—the Buddha said the most difficult thing for a human being to do is to stay still. Our emotions are what drive us to action, so learning to stay still in the face of them is against our instincts.

Secondly, it brings into question everything we think about how our emotions operate. We usually believe that other people and what happens in our lives cause the emotions we experience, and we don't see that this belief actually disempowers us. It puts our emotional life at the whim of whomever we happen to be with and the situations we find ourselves in.

Because staying still in the face of emotions is so difficult, the meditation tradition has developed hundreds of ways to train ourselves to do this. This is the essence of meditation: simply learning to stay still, and then discovering that when you do, your mind and emotions will naturally balance themselves. This happens every time, and brings us to the next step in dealing with a powerful emotion.

Watching emotions

Watching emotions takes practice. **The POW! Technique** is a quick, clean way to discharge the effect of emotions like anger and frees you from bottling things up in your body. However, it doesn't lead to understanding how emotions work—what they are, what causes them, why they are so strong, and what purpose they serve. So it's a skillful short-term solution. Watching emotions is a longer-term project.

The purpose of emotions

Scientists are just beginning to understand the purpose of emotions such as joy, anger, sadness and grief (the meditation tradition, of course, has made a detailed study of emotions over thousands of years). These emotions appear to be hardwired into our makeup and each has served a primary function in our evolution. For example, sadness causes you to disengage and conserve energy when there is a loss. Anger is very energetic and moves you to protect yourself and those you love, and to keep going if you have been blocked. Fear keeps you alert and joy is the release of energy after it has been built up—when something has come to fruition. It brings us together and creates social bonds, cooperation and altruism.

However, the first three of these emotions: sadness, anger and fear, don't always feel like that at the time! This is because we no longer live under the conditions for which these emotions were designed. In the wild they would be quick, immediate responses to actual physical threats or situations that affected the wellbeing of the body. Once the situation was over, the body would relax again. The reason they have become so difficult to deal with is because of our conscious, thinking mind.

The reason for emotional conflict

Whether something has *actually* happened, or whether we *think* it has happened, makes no difference to our bodies. Thinking about something creates exactly the same emotional response as the actual physical situation. This is how all emotional conflict arises—our bodies respond to thoughts about what might or might not happen, and not to the actual physical situation for which they were designed. This emotional conflict then causes the residual feelings and moods to lodge in our bodies.

In the wild something actually happens—there is no time to muse over what may or may not happen, because by that time you would probably be dead! When you are faced with real physical danger there is often no strong emotional response—you just react. Any emotion you experience at a time like this is very clear and direct. Some scientists believe that a true emotion only lasts for a few seconds and I totally agree with them.

The conflict comes later when you have time to think about what happened and you start to experience the conflict and pain which characterise many emotions. This is because your conscious mind has kicked in and started to construct a story about what has happened, linking it to your past experience and memories.

In cities we have plenty of time to mull over things and create stories about who did what to whom, and we don't realise that our bodies are responding to these thoughts in the same way they would to real, physical events in the wild. However, because they are thoughts, the physical cue that the threat is over does not happen, so our bodies don't get the chance to let go of the emotion and move on.

What were quick, healthy responses to real situations become stuck in the body and very unhealthy. The normal discharge through appropriate action cannot then happen. We aren't able to distinguish between a real threat and our stories about what is happening.

What complicates this further is that so much of our interaction is now through language rather than action, and our bodies and emotions were designed for action. For example, in our society we now attack verbally rather than physically. If a person in a position of power is threatened by someone else, he or she attacks through words or moves politically to make the other person's life and career more difficult. And at home, words can be used in extremely painful ways because family members know each other's weak spots so well.

Social constraints mean that when someone suffers like this, they can't punch out or yell—they have to literally swallow whatever they are feeling. This then lodges in the body and forms a knot, so they start to construct stories in their mind about what has happened.

For example, if someone is verbally attacked at work, it feels as though they have been in a life-threatening situation, as though their entire career and identity are under attack, so their bodies are on full alert. However, physically they haven't been attacked and they are not in a life-threatening situation.

Here then, is the emotional conflict they suffer. What they feel is not in touch with what has actually happened. Because the thought of losing a position is threatening to their financial situation and their view of themselves—their *identity*—they respond emotionally in the same way as if their bodies were in a life-threatening situation. *Not being able to distinguish between real physical threats and what we think happened is the source of all emotional conflict.*

Meditation deals with this kind of conflict. The Buddha described being free from the underlying anxiety generated by the conscious mind as seeing all the snakes turning back into pieces of rope. You can distinguish clearly between events that have actually happened and the stories generated by your thoughts about what may or may not have happened.

How to observe emotions in everyday life

The process for observing emotions in everyday life is an extension of the **Three C Technique**. Firstly and most importantly (and possibly the most difficult thing to do) is to acknowledge and accept what you are feeling.

Accepting what you feel (Catch the moment)

This is the step of **Catching the moment**, and it can be difficult for a couple of reasons. We are trained not to act on strong emotions so we feel guilt about having them in the first place. Nice people simply don't have these kinds of feelings. So we have to give up being nice and remember that our bodies are not nice—they are real!

Secondly, these emotions are often so unconscious we don't even know they are there. Me, angry? I'm never angry! Or, I've never been jealous in all my life! So staying still in your chair and allowing yourself to feel the agitation, anxiety, anger or other conflict in your body is the first step. Give yourself time and space to stay with the emotion, just accepting it, and naming it so that you can say to yourself, as best you can, exactly what you are feeling.

Just letting it be (Clear the space)

The next step is to **Clear the space** and this is where you use meditation. Instead of trying to work out the cause of the emotion, "expressing" or getting rid of it, just let it be there. Set yourself up in a formal meditation posture, gently rock from side to side until your body finds its own balance point, take a deep breath into your belly and sigh, and then open your mind to all the sounds around you.

You need to establish your balance, physically, emotionally and mentally, because this is the only way you can release your mind from the stories: the "ifs", "buts" and "maybes" surrounding what you are feeling; the "awfullising" and "catastrophising". Let yourself focus on your breath, a bodyscan, mantra or visualisation—whatever your favourite and most effective form of meditation is—until you feel yourself reach your balance point.

Then space will open up in your mind and body. Instead of incessant inner conversation and the physical tension which accompanies it, you will feel your body open as the muscles relax and loosen and your mind clears.

Finding the focus of the emotion in your body (Change the habit)

Now you are ready to **Change the habit**. Once you have established your balance, start to explore the actual physical sensations in your body. See if you can find the focus of the emotion; where the tension or agitation is localised. Stay with this feeling and explore it.

You have now moved your focus away from your thoughts and stories around the emotions, to the actual sensation your body is experiencing. You can now just watch it. If it helps, try to describe what the sensation looks and feels like. What shape would it be? What colour is it? After your meditation session you might even like to draw it.

Now that you are dealing with what your body is actually experiencing you can do something about it. When you listen to your body it often knows what to do, you just need to get out of the way. So you might find that your body starts breathing deeply. If this happens, help it by joining in—breathe directly into the focus of tension, into the knot. You might visualise what is happening and create a picture of what is needed to let the knot go, and work with your body in this way.

Or you might find that your body begins to shake involuntarily. If this happens, don't be afraid of losing control. Meditation provides a safe boundary for whatever happens, so let it happen. It will stop as soon as as soon as you stop meditating. This is one of the quickest ways for the body to release the tension that has been locked up and stored from emotions you experience.

An emotional toolkit

I have used this technique with many people referred to me due to severe trauma in their lives, or who find they are caught in a habitual, painful emotion. With meditation they can become aware of the sensations they are experiencing, know exactly where they are located, and release the knots which have formed there. They are able to move past the images which have become fixed in their mind, so can let go of them and, through being able to come back to their bodies and open to what they are experiencing right now, balance themselves emotionally, trust their own bodies, and find peace. Importantly, it's something they can do alone once they know how, and it's always there when they need it.

Without exception, once their focus moved from their minds to their bodies, they felt the trauma or emotion begin to release. The relief in each case was palpable. The same principle applies to all the usual conflicts—the meditative emotional toolkit can help enormously in dealing with the day-to-day emotional wear and tear we all experience.

Instructions for letting go of emotions

Catch the moment

Acknowledge and accept what you are feeling.

Sit in your chair and allow yourself to feel the agitation, anxiety, anger or other conflict in your body.

Give it a name so that you can say to yourself, as best you can, exactly what you are feeling.

Clear the space

Instead of trying to deal with the emotion, trying to work out its cause, or "express" or get rid of it, just let it be there.

Set yourself up in a formal meditation posture, then gently rock from side to side until your body finds its own balance point. Run through the Bodycheck, take a deep breath into your belly and sigh, then open your mind to all the sounds around you.

Focus on your meditation exercise.

Notice the space open up in your mind and body.

Change the habit

Try to find where the emotion (tension or agitation) is located in your body. Stay with this feeling and explore it. You can now just watch it as a sensation in your body instead of being caught in the stories around it.

Describe to yourself what the sensation looks and feels like. What shape is it? What colour is it? *(After your meditation session you might try to draw it.)*

You might find that your body starts breathing deeply. If this happens, help it on its way by joining in—breathe directly into the focus of tension, into the knot.

You might visualise what is happening and create a picture of what is needed to let the knot go.

If your body begins to shake involuntarily, don't be afraid of losing control. It will stop as soon as you stop meditating. This is one of the quickest ways for the body to release the tension that has been locked up and stored from the emotions you experience.

The next chapter explores how to recognise unhealthy states of mind and cultivate healthy states so you can maintain your balance in daily life.

Chapter 9: The weather patterns of the mind

Recognising when the mind is in a healthy, balanced state and when it is in an unhealthy state is one of the most important things that can be learned from meditation.

When your mind and body are deeply balanced, it is an exquisitely blissful experience. Different people respond to it in different ways. Some experience a sense of awe or transcendence from which they draw a deep feeling of inspiration. Others experience it as a profound connection with the environment and others feel a sense of union with God or deep peace.

All of these experiences are expressions of what it is like to be deeply balanced. This is the natural state of our minds and bodies and we feel a sense of unity, bliss and clarity each time we touch it in meditation. In everyday life, we usually don't experience it because we are so preoccupied with our thoughts and emotions, but this safe place in our minds is open, spacious and expansive, beyond all judgements of good and bad.

From this deeply balanced state you begin to see that your mind and life move in patterns and cycles, just like weather patterns. Recognising when the mind is in a healthy, balanced state and when it is in an unhealthy state is one of the most important things that can be learned from meditation. Your state of mind determines the way you feel about yourself and how you look at the world around you. It affects your physical health and your relationships with others.

This chapter explores the cycles of the mind, different states of mind and how to recognise and sustain a healthy state of mind.

Seeing the weather patterns of your mind

Imagine the kinds of emotions you would have if you genuinely believed that you controlled the weather. Each sunny day (presuming you liked sunny days) would bring elation and possibly a drunken sense of power as you believed that you created it. Then when it became cloudy, raining and a thunderstorm appeared over the horizon you would be shattered. You would have completely failed. Elation would be followed by depression. Up and down your emotions would go, totally at the mercy of the weather patterns, without you being able to do anything about it.

Believing that we control, or should control, our states of mind is exactly the same and leads to the same result. It guarantees that we don't come to see and understand how our minds actually work because we are looking in the wrong place.

An unhealthy state of mind is not caused by "cloudy weather"—by thinking about things, feeling tired or even a bit annoyed. An unhealthy state is caused by our *reaction* to this. For example, if it is raining and cold and we are dressed for a sunny day because we believe that, as we control the weather, this aberration of rain shouldn't be happening— well it's not hard to guess the result.

We know how to avoid getting physically ill by adjusting our behaviour and clothing to the climate, eating well and washing. Keeping the mind in a reasonably healthy state is no different; however, it is impossible if we are blinded by wanting things to be perfect and believing that we control it. Without any emotional training whatsoever, we are expected to control our minds.

As we move from trying to fix how we feel and control what our minds are doing to learning how to establish a calm state, we can accept how we feel without needing to do anything about it. We can then watch, and discover what our thoughts and emotions actually do.

The cycles of the mind

As each day has its cycle and the seasons move in a particular cycle each year, your mind and body also have their cycles, and meditation provides the space and calm to watch them and learn how they operate. Meditation retreats provide the ideal environment to experience this because you are not so busy that you don't have time to notice. In retreat you can feel how the day changes as it moves from early morning to late afternoon and then into night, because you notice how your body actually responds to these changes. You can watch changes of light during the day, and the way animals and birds behave at different times of the day.

As you notice these physical changes, you become aware that your mind is also changing and responding. At certain times of the day it is fresh and full of energy, and at others it is quiet and naturally seeks to turn in.

We usually believe that we should be marching ever onwards and upwards, bright, full of energy and endlessly busy. And so we plough on, driving ourselves harder and faster, without having any idea of how our emotions work, or how to look after ourselves emotionally, or even that we need to.

When you watch the cycles of the day and your body's responses, it becomes obvious that this is unsustainable. There comes a time when the energy is spent, and your mind and body need to restore themselves. The law that anything which goes up in the physical world must come down also applies in our emotional world. Our emotions naturally move up and down: so whenever you have been "up" the next move will be to come "down" to restore the energy.

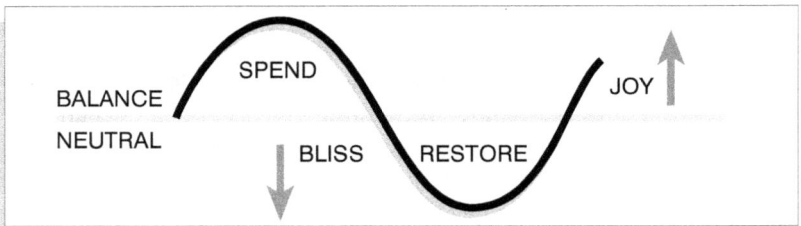

In developing a meditation practice you come to know the neutral balance point between "up" and "down" (illustrated above), and you can become aware of the process of spending and restoring energy. Knowing this balance point—the stillness of meditation—and knowing how to get there enables you to keep your emotional balance.

When you become aware of these patterns you can respond to them instead of trying to control them. You can become aware when the energy is there to move quickly, and act skillfully and efficiently. You also know when and how to turn in, to give your mind and body time to restore themselves.

States of mind—keeping your balance

When the mind is balanced, so is the body. In a healthy state, mind and body are connected. When you become unbalanced, the mind and body are disconnected—you are stuck in an emotion and starting to cling to the ideas associated with it, believing you should stay either "up" or "down". If you cling to an idea of what should be happening you are stuck. This creates an unhealthy state of mind, because the mind becomes rigid.

A teenage boy suffering from anxiety had no idea how to describe it, so I asked him to draw it. Without hesitation he drew a jagged line with sharp spikes in it.

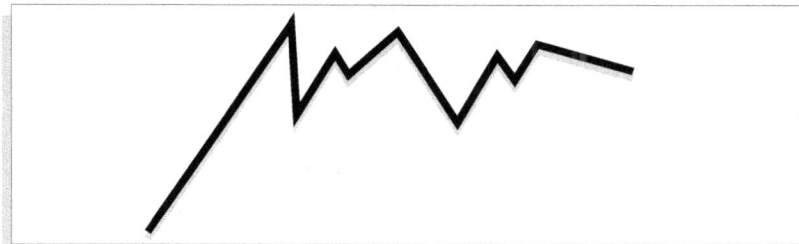

This jagged line perfectly describes what it feels like to be stuck and unbalanced. After he meditated, I again asked him to draw his feelings.

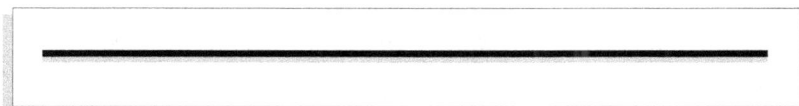

This simple, straight line describes how he felt after meditating—resting in a balanced state.

Flexible and open or rigid and closed

A healthy state of mind is flexible and open. It can be sharp, brilliant, clear and totally focused or it can be soft and warm, or spacious and connected with everything. When the state of mind is unhealthy it can be rigid and closed, scattered and distracted, or too loose and floppy. It is closed to the senses, closed to listening to others and to new ideas—to anything that requires a change of mind. You literally get caught in a closed loop, going round and round in a cage of thought and emotion, which is completely disconnected from your senses and the direct experience of your body.

You veer towards increasing agitation, busyness and anxiety, pushing harder to make what you think should be happening happen, or towards the other side of the spectrum of losing interest and energy, becoming bored and lethargic, and eventually feeling a bit depressed. (These emotional stages are outlined in detail in Chapter 13.)

Recognising states of mind

Through meditating you can become friends with your states of mind as you come to know them and see how they operate. You don't have to battle them—as you don't battle the sea or weather. You know when the mind is still and calm, and when it is thinking. You know when you are open to what you are actually experiencing and when you are stuck on an idea of what should be happening. It's not whether our minds are sharp and bright or a bit dull and tired that determines whether it is an unhealthy state. *It's whether we find it difficult to accept what is happening and want it to be different.*

The moment you accept whatever your mind is doing you are calm, concentrated, connected with your body and senses and in a healthy state of mind. The moment you start to worry about what is happening, trying to fix it or wanting it to be otherwise, you are caught in an unhealthy state. It's as quick as that—which means that as soon as you become aware you are stuck on trying to avoid whatever you are feeling, you are able to shift immediately to a healthy state of mind. *Acceptance of what is happening* is the key to maintaining this.

Sustaining a healthy state of mind

When we learn to recognise the health or otherwise of our state of mind it is possible to deliberately keep our minds in a good state. We often feel a bit embarrassed about the idea of consciously feeding a good state—we feel it should somehow look after itself. However, it's surprising how much we actually *feed an unhealthy state*—we hold it there, trying to sort it out, talking about it with everyone else over endless coffees or beers, and worrying about it, without realising that in doing all this we are actually maintaining it. So trying to fix an unhealthy state is a lost cause—it only increases being stuck in it. The focus remains on that state so it can't change.

By meditating you can accept the state of mind; *just watching* brings you immediately back into a state of balance. There is a space created in which you can feel unstuck from that state. The worry stops as you reconnect with your body and feelings. There is then space in the mind to be aware of everything else you are feeling. What you were concerned about takes its place among everything else—the broader context reappears and this change of perspective opens up the quality of completeness.

It's exactly as though you were focused on a particular cloud in the sky and then shifted your perspective to become aware of the whole sky itself. Thoughts are exactly like clouds in the sky; they can be wispy and light or heavy and dark. They come and go. The reason clouds don't dominate our lives and cause us anxiety is because we know their patterns and we see the sky in which they form, which is constant.

Meditation allows us to see that our minds operate in exactly the same way. To maintain a healthy state of mind you simply need to keep in touch with the space in which thoughts come and go. Then it is possible to see that they *do* come and go and that they are not permanent. Every time you meditate you touch that space—the open sky of the mind. And every time you touch that space you restore the balance of your mind and body because thoughts take their place as simply part of your mind instead of feeling like they are the whole mind.

Observing the state of mind before acting

With the balance restored your mind is complete. The space is in view as well as the thoughts, and your mind is in a healthy state. As this state of mind becomes increasingly familiar it can become the reference point for all the states you experience. This means there is a place you can rest and observe what is happening.

Before going into any situation you can use this ability to assess whether you are in a healthy or unhealthy state. This can be crucial to determining the outcome, because if you are in a healthy state you won't bring any conflict or unrealistic expectations to the situation. You are emotionally balanced, so will not lose your balance when you move and are less likely to become caught if there are unhealthy emotions around, so at least one person is not adding to the confusion.

A good surfer always examines the sea before going in to the surf, checking out the weather, watching how the waves are breaking and where the currents and rips are. We can pay the same kind of respect to our mind by observing its patterns, and seeing how the waves of our emotions are moving before going into important situations. This will definitely help to ensure we aren't swept away in a wave, or caught in an emotional rip or undertow.

How to recognise states of mind

In Chapter 3 I explained how to tune your meditations by becoming aware of how tightly or loosely you are holding your body and mind. This is the key to becoming aware of your states of mind, because as you become too tight, you are moving into an agitated state of mind, and as you become too loose, your state of mind is becoming lethargic. Your meditation sessions are the best time to come to know your states of mind because you need the calm of meditation to have the space to step back and see them. However, what can make it difficult is that we are so used to living with unhealthy emotions that we don't even know they are there.

For example, it took me a long time to see how much I pushed myself because I was used to living in a slightly agitated and worried state. This came from being a concert pianist—the pressure of having to be on call, doing concerts, have new pieces ready quickly and keeping a very high standard. This state is so normal in that world that no-one would ever consider it unhealthy. However, my body would rebel and I would catch colds and the flu fairly regularly. Again, this was "normal".

It was only after learning what it was like to maintain healthy states of mind in my meditation sessions that I began to feel the damage I was doing to my body, and it became apparent what the long-term consequences would be. I discovered that I could achieve everything much more efficiently and effectively without having to push so hard and drive myself into this agitated and worried state.

So when you sit down to meditate and find it's not going where you think it should because your mind is still busy making important decisions and worrying about what needs to be done—*there's your state of mind*. There's nothing wrong with your meditation. In fact it's going very well. You have the space to see your state of mind, instead of it driving your life.

If you believe that the meditation is not going well, and that it would be better to stop and *do* all those things, then you're stuck. You are caught in the closed loop of your thoughts. If you allow your thoughts to stop the meditation and act on them, you will be moving from an unbalanced state and this will drive you to becoming totally unbalanced. Staying with the meditation and *watching* this state will not only balance you, but bring you to the point where you can see and feel how to act from that state of balance.

You don't have to be deeply balanced to see your states of mind. Becoming physically still, relaxing a little and letting your mind slow down is enough. You are then in a good position to be aware of how you feel, see what your emotions are doing, and so see your state of mind.

Surprisingly, sometimes we don't recognise when we are in a good state of mind because it can be fairly quiet. If you are unused to being without anxiety or agitation it can take a while to become aware of your senses when they are not over-stimulated. Again, by staying with the meditation you are learning to just watch, feel the constant play of your senses, and see that this quiet and seemingly ordinary state is actually a vivid, healthy state of mind.

Of course, moments of wild exuberance where you relish the living vitality of your senses, or when you collapse into a state of complete rest, are also wonderfully healthy states of mind. What keeps them healthy is the awareness you bring to them, which keeps you in touch with your body. The aim of maintaining healthy states of mind is to be open to the vibrancy and beauty of the life around us and within us and so lead richer, more fulfilling lives.

Meditations for recognising states of mind and maintaining healthy states

Start by doing one or two loosening exercises to look after your body. Then, when you sit down to meditate, balance yourself physically by doing the Rocking exercise and Bodycheck. Having established your physical balance point, you can then move to your chosen meditation to balance yourself mentally and emotionally. From this state of balance you will be able to recognise your state of mind, because you have a reference point.

You can also use your meditation to maintain a healthy state of mind. The Nourishing Breath Meditation (see Chapter 4) is particularly good for feeding yourself emotionally and keeping your mind in a good state.

Watching the breath
Watching your breath is one of the best meditations for recognising your states of mind, because every emotion, thought, and state of mind has its own breathing pattern.

A good exercise to demonstrate this is to deliberately breathe very quickly and forcefully, keeping the breath high in your chest. Keep this up for ten breaths.

Then stop immediately and notice how you feel. What are the sensations in your body? Which emotions are you feeling, and where are they in your body? What does your state of mind feel like?

Then do the Instant Calm Breath

1. Breathe out with a little sigh.

2. Take a deep breath in, just to where it is comfortable, feeling the movement of your abdomen.

3. Now hold your breath for a while—just as long as is comfortable for you.

4. Finally, and this is the key, breathe out as slowly and smoothly as you are able.

Notice how you feel and compare this with the previous exercise. Which emotions are you feeling now, and where are they in your body? What does your state of mind feel like?

This exercise clearly demonstrates the difference between the two states and you will see how quickly you can change an emotion and state of mind.

Along with your observations in meditation, you can use the open, balanced state of *just watching* (awareness) to listen to what your family and friends tell you about yourself and your states of mind. They are usually only too keen and have a good perspective because it is easier to see someone else than yourself, so use those moments as a meditation to open up and listen.

The next chapter explores how you can use informal meditations to keep yourself in a light meditative state—a healthy state of mind.

Chapter 10: Informal meditations

Informal meditations ensure that you stay in touch with your senses and don't get lost in your thoughts. You approach everything as though it were the first time because, in actual fact, it is.

Many things we do in our lives become so repetitive that we don't even notice them any more—this means we spend an awful lot of our lives in a semi-hypnotic trance, unaware of what we are doing. How often have you driven home and not known how you arrived? Totally lost in the world of our thoughts, worries, hopes, fears and plans, we completely lose touch with our senses and the reality of our lives.

There is a saying in the Zen tradition: "Zen mind—beginner's mind", which has a profound meaning. It points to the fact that nothing in life is ever an exact repetition—there is always a change, no matter how similar two events might appear. When we name something, we assume we know what it is, and that we have seen it, so we stop looking. We also assume that everything with the same name is exactly the same. But, of course, it isn't.

So being in touch with your senses requires giving up assuming; this is what is meant by having a beginner's mind. You approach everything as though it were the first time because, in actual fact, it is.

With informal meditations you can use the routines of your daily life to hold your focus on your senses, keeping your mind with what you are doing and therefore keeping yourself mentally and emotionally balanced.

This chapter outlines a range of simple informal meditations, which allow you to keep in touch with this healthy state.

Keeping yourself connected

Informal meditations, along with Spot Meditations, are ideally suited to help you find your balance no matter what you are doing, so that your work, actions and thinking become more efficient. They are also the best way to learn how to "change gears" skillfully and smoothly.

Instead of pushing ahead, doggedly ploughing on, becoming busier and more frantic, you can keep your external balance by moving to your inner balance point—that point of stillness you touch each time you meditate. Then you can move back to what you need to do, having refreshed your mind and emotions.

It is therefore possible to live in a happy state and keep yourself emotionally healthy no matter what you are experiencing.

How to meditate informally

You can turn any task into a meditation, especially those everyday, repetitive tasks that form the background ritual in our lives. Some examples are showering, cleaning your teeth, going to the toilet and having a cup of tea or coffee.

By turning such tasks into a short meditation you achieve a light meditative state. This state is both useful in your everyday life and extremely beneficial for your mental and physical health, because it is alert, open to the senses, calm, and free from destructive emotions.

To meditate informally you simply choose an activity, slow it down slightly, focus on your physical sensations and keep your mind with the actual experience of what is happening.

Here are the five steps in the process:

1. Choose an activity.
2. Slow it down slightly, so that it becomes a smooth action, unhurried.
3. Focus on the physical sensations (touch, taste, sight, smell, sound) so that your thinking goes into the background.
4. Keep your mind with the action—bring your mind back when it wanders (for example, when eating, eat).
5. Notice what happens.

If you compare these steps with the four steps of the meditation technique itself you will see that you are following the same process:

1. Relax the body.
2. Focus the mind on a meditation object.
3. Notice thoughts when the mind wanders.
4. Then let them go into the background by bringing your mind back to the object.

The difference is that *you are using whatever you are doing as the meditation object*. This is why you need to slightly slow it down—no-one else will notice—so you can move your mind away from your thoughts to focus on the sense experience, rather than relying on habit to get the task done.

Then you follow the same process as for formal meditation: you focus on the object—just doing this will calm your mind. When you start to think about things again, notice what you are thinking about, then bring your mind back to keep it there with what you are doing.

Benefits of informal meditations

Informal meditations are very effective when you are too agitated, tired or busy to settle down for a more formal meditation. They can be used anywhere at any time, so are an extremely simple way to incorporate the habit of meditating into your everyday life.

They are also a great way to approach the repetitive tasks we all have to do every day of our lives. Turning such tasks into informal meditations keeps them alive, interesting and fresh because they can be used productively to keep your mind in a clear, healthy state.

Examples of informal meditations

Eating

Eating food is something we do a number of times every day, and it can be anything from a boring, tiresome necessity or ritual through to an obsession, drama or celebration. However, it's quite a discovery to realise how little we actually *eat* when we are eating.

Repeatedly in our courses, when students eat something as an informal meditation, they are very surprised to experience what it is like to be totally in touch with the sensation of eating. The fact we usually remain concentrated on our thoughts and pay very little attention to the sense experience of food is why many people eat too much—they hardly register the effect, so can be left feeling hungry because their mind is so disconnected from their body.

In our introductory courses we offer people a piece of fruit: either a grape, raisin, piece of orange or mandarin, or good quality chocolate to use as an informal eating meditation.

Instructions for informal eating meditation

Hold the piece of food in your hand—feel its texture, notice its colour, shape and smell.

Then put it in your mouth and hold it there for a while, noticing the feel of the food on your tongue, the taste in your mouth and the effect this has on your body.

Then suck it and explore the sensations.

When you are ready, bite into it and see if there is any change in taste and texture.

Then chew and swallow. Again notice all the sensations as you do this.

When we use food as meditation in our courses and retreats, people calm down and become more in touch with their bodies as they explore the sensual experience of eating. It is completely absorbing when you notice all the details of colour and shape, touch, taste, smell and texture, and even the sound of eating.

Smelling a plant

The other object I bring to class for an informal meditation is a very old-fashioned plant. I choose this plant because the smell is so complex. It ranges from very sweet through to a medicinal menthol eucalyptus to quite bitter, so it really opens up the sense of smell. I ask people to hold it while noticing the colour, feeling and texture, then rub a little between their hands and bury their noses in it. It's a very rich, full-on experience.

Everyone is so puzzled by this plant that they become totally absorbed in the experience. Because it is not well known—only two people have ever recognised it—they are kept puzzled, and this keeps them right there with the experience. So I would like to keep it that way and not disclose the name of this mysterious plant!

Giving yourself time to stop and smell a plant or flower, or the air in a park or by the sea, can be a wonderful discovery and makes a very effective informal meditation.

Visual objects

You can use any visual object as an informal meditation, choosing something that catches your eye and focusing in on it for a few seconds, allowing your mind to rest in the shape, colour and texture of the object.

Instructions for informal visual object meditation

Let your eyes rest for a moment on something which takes your interest. Soften your eyes to let them rest on the object rather than examining it.

Notice the colours, shapes and textures.

Allow yourself to "feel" the effect of it.
Close your eyes for a moment and see if the image is still there.
Is it the same as the object or are there differences?

Light

Reflected light has a soft quality to it and watching it on the leaves of trees or water immediately takes your mind away from its busyness and allows your body to relax and your mind to become still.

Instructions for informal meditation on light

There are three ways to do this:

1. Notice the reflection of light on the leaves of a tree and let your mind rest on the light. Then let your eyes soften as you allow your mind to become absorbed in the light.
2. Light reflected on water makes a beautiful meditation object. Whenever you are by the sea, notice the shimmering effect of sunlight on the water, or the stream of moonlight moving across the sea. Again, allow your mind to rest in the light, absorbing it. This meditation can be done with any body of water.
3. The light in the sky at dawn and dusk is ideal for meditation. At this time of day the light is soft and diffuse, and moves your mind away from feeling tight and closed to being clear and open.

One student, looking for a place to meditate during the day, decided to stop at a parking bay on the road when she drove home from work, and found it was an ideal place to watch the sunset each night. This became her daily meditation.

When you go for a walk or are sitting outside, and find your mind going over its usual conversations and concerns, meditating on light can literally lighten your mind. It brings a physical feeling of "lightening up", and also a quality of light in your mind as the thoughts open to reveal the clear, open, vibrant space behind them. This quality of light can flow through your whole body, so that you are filled with a blissful feeling of radiance.

Wind and air

Another lovely informal meditation is to watch the movement of trees or grass in the wind and to feel the air moving over your skin. It can have an extremely soothing effect on your mind and body.

Instructions for informal meditation on wind or air

Allow your mind to rest on the swaying of the trees or grass, and open your body to the feeling of the movement of air across your skin. It can feel as though you are being brushed with silk, and embraced by the air and space around you.

Sounds

Sound is a wonderful way to meditate informally as we are constantly bathed in it. It's an extremely effective way to take your mind out of thought and let it rest in the sheer sensation of any sounds around you.

Instructions for informal sound meditation

Allow your mind to open up and listen to all the sounds around you—absolutely everything.

Listen out in all directions, allowing everything to come into your awareness. This means that you stop focusing on any one sound in particular, and become aware of the background wash of sound which surrounds you.

If you are inside, start by listening to all the sounds in the room. Then move to listening to all the sounds in the building.

Then open up to all the sounds outside and listen out as far as you possibly can. You will find you can let your mind rest in the sensation of sound itself, as though there is a huge sphere of sound which holds your mind still.

A wonderful place to meditate on sound is at the beach, listening to the sounds of the waves; you can reach a point where you hear and feel the waves through your entire body. You can do the same thing with the sound of wind—especially the sound of the wind in trees.

You will discover the ripple of sensations through your body as it responds to the sound. These sensations are always there, but usually we only notice them when the sound is so loud that the jolt to our body shocks us. One sad cost of living a busy city life is that we become desensitised to the wash of sensations constantly passing through our bodies, particularly those responding to light and sound. Over the years, lighting has become much brighter and music much louder to catch your attention.

The price of relying on light and sound to be extra bright and extra loud is that for the rest of the time we tend to feel dull and empty, or worse, nothing at all. I believe that this loss of contact with the inner sensations of the body causes a great deal of depression.

The informal meditations on light and sound are a wonderful way to re-sensitise yourself and discover what a rich world of sensation is moving in a constant stream through your body. These sensations are your life, and the aim of meditation is to make you aware of just how rich and vibrant life is.

Music

Music lends itself perfectly to meditating informally. Many of us become used to music as a constant background noise—it's just there and we don't really listen to it. To meditate on music you do need to listen. Like all meditation, the more you focus on the object, the better it is.

Really good music is designed to literally "touch" you. It can play the body like an instrument: getting your energies moving, thrilling and inspiring you and blowing the top of your head off! It can stimulate your mind and clear your head. It can touch your heart, and also satisfy your gut feelings. It can also caress and stroke your whole body and send tingles up your spine.

It's an exploration to feel your body resonating to the sounds.

Sit comfortably or lie down to listen.

Let your mind open to the music, resting in it, following the music.

See if you can follow your body's reactions to the sounds as the music resonates through your body.

Notice when you wander off to something else, and bring your mind back.

Walking and other daily activities

Walking, preparing food for cooking, gardening and many of the things we do to relax can be turned into informal meditations by bringing your mind to the actual sense experience. Instead of hoping to relax while your mind continues its normal chatter, you can enhance the experience by consciously using it to relax your body, calm your mind and refresh yourself.

Instructions for informal walking meditations

As you walk, develop a sense of embracing the ground with your feet.

At the beach, walking in bare feet on damp sand will slow you down a little and bring you to focus on the feeling of your feet on the sand. The walking meditation also becomes a form of foot massage. Feel the sand shaping around your foot and moving between your toes.

(This is an ancient Chinese remedy for healing nervous disorders.)

Watching clouds in the sky

Finally, watching clouds in the sky is an effective way to remember how thoughts work and immediately dissolve the power they can have.

Watch clouds forming, changing shape and dissolving, and notice the sky between them. You will start to feel this process in your mind as you open to the space between your thoughts.

Checklist for informal meditations

After meditating informally it can be useful to run through the checklist to see how it went.

- Have your thoughts slowed down a bit, or were there times when you felt completely free from them?
- Does your mind feel calmer, more settled and less scattered or busy?
- Do you feel more connected with your body and what you are doing?
- Is there a bit more space around you so that you don't feel so tight and hemmed in?
- Are your senses more alive and open—brighter and clearer—and do you feel more in touch with them?

Taking a moment to check these things helps you become aware of the subtle changes that occur in your mind and body as you meditate. It provides a template of what to look for each time you meditate, and informal meditations are a good way to do this because you are still engaged in the things you normally do. You notice that you feel a little calmer, more content with what you are doing, more in touch with your senses and your whole body. These are signs that you have become balanced; that your mind and body are working together instead of being in conflict.

The next chapter explains how a retreat can deepen and enhance your meditation practice, by providing conditions free from the pressures of daily life.

Chapter 11: Retreat

The more you become aware of the cycles of your mind and body, the happier your life will become.

A retreat is a rich and rewarding way to complement and help sustain your meditation practice. In retreat, you are free from your usual daily concerns so have time to completely focus on and deepen your meditation experience—you are in an environment which has been specifically created to support meditation. Many people discover how precious it is to have this space—to be free from the roles they normally have to play in social relationships and the conversations they habitually engage in.

In retreat you are free to explore aspects of your life which are usually neglected. You also have the opportunity to reconnect with your body and the natural environment surrounding you. This is an incredible relief because when you open up to the continuous, vibrant stream of sensations coursing through your body, your mind returns to its foundation of calm, clear awareness.

Opening up to your senses

Retreat provides a safe way to relax your mind and body, so you can open up to *all* of your senses, not just the dominant ones (for most people sight is dominant). This is a key practice in retreat.

Normally our lives involve thinking most of the time: planning for the future and setting goals, recalling and reinforcing memories from the past, thinking about other people's experiences and comparing them with our own ideas and views. We are constantly naming and judging things as mine or yours, good and bad. The media is also ever present––the internet, newspapers, television and radio all stimulate thinking.

During retreat the aim is to shift from thinking to sensing. Your thinking doesn't disappear, it just shifts to the background and you have the opportunity to become fully aware of your body. Often, when you do become more aware of the real needs of your body, you feel quite tired. Many people are sleep deprived, so their bodies are not getting the rest they need to fully rejuvenate their energies. During the first part of a retreat, you may need to just accept that you feel tired and allow yourself to rest as much as possible. This is the quickest way to restore your energies, and if you are doing a retreat over a weekend you will usually find that after a third of the way through, you are fresher and more energised.

The cycles of nature

A retreat also provides the opportunity to become aware of the rhythm of each day and night—the cycles of nature. This will bring you in touch with the natural rhythms and cycles of your own mind and body. You become aware of the changes in your body as it responds to the cycles of morning, noon and evening. You will notice your senses opening up to the night, which has its own rhythm as it moves from sunset to sunrise. Feeling your body responding to this change is one of the most profoundly moving experiences you can have on this planet.

The more you become aware of the cycles of your own mind and body, the more efficiently you can work with them, and the happier your life will become. Retreat provides the foundation for you to experience this and then you can begin to integrate it with your daily life.

Retreat exercises

There are a number of exercises to help quickly establish the calm, balanced alertness that forms the foundation of all retreat work.

Building your sense awareness

Here are some simple ways to open to your senses while in retreat. Practise bringing your mind back to the immediate physical experience.

Open up to nature by watching the changes of light during the day.

Watch the sunrise and sunset and feel the effects on your body.

Notice the colours of flowers and plants—observe the details in the natural world around you.

Notice movement around you: watch clouds come and go, trees and grass blowing in the wind.

Open your mind to all the sounds around you—letting them resonate through your mind and body.

Listen to the sounds of day and night, particularly the birds and animals.

Hear the birds waking in the morning and settling down at night.

Listen for the crickets and frogs in the paddocks at night.

Smell the different scents during the day.

Notice how things smell differently in the early morning, at midday and in the evening.

Remember that your whole skin is your sense of touch.

Feel the changes in temperature on your skin and feel the wind, sun and rain on your skin.

Become aware of the response of your skin to everything around you.

Taste the air and the objects around you.

Notice any changes in your body as night approaches.

See if your body responds to these changes and sounds.

Naming the senses

A good exercise for retreat is to become aware of which sense you are using at any particular time.

You can do this by moving away from thinking about what you are doing or what your mind is focused on to just becoming aware of which sense you are using.

Some people find it useful to silently name the sense they are using. So if you are looking at something, say to yourself "Seeing". If hearing something, say "Hearing"; if smelling, say "Smelling"; if tasting, say "Tasting" and if touching, say "Touching".

Practise this on walks. See how much you can open to what is around you—instead of thinking about it or something else.

Find out which sense you keep coming back to, the one you rely on most.

Turning ordinary activities into meditations

Retreat is an excellent time to turn daily activities into meditations (see also Chapter 10).

Practise eating with full awareness, tasting each mouthful of food.

Notice the feel of ordinary things on your skin, for example, when you are showering, getting dressed or washing dishes. Cultivate awareness of the skin over your whole body.

Practise walking just to walk. With each step you take, feel the earth with your feet; embrace the earth with your feet.

Bring your breathing into line with your walking: two steps (breathing in); two steps (breathing out)—or whatever suits you.

Keeping your eyes closed, hold different objects and try to identify them by listening, touching, tasting and smelling.

Massage your hands, face and feet, particularly in the evening.

Opening your mind

As your mind opens on retreat, you will feel more spacious as you begin to include what is around you into your awareness, instead of blocking it out as we normally do (which causes us to feel small and tight—we literally shrink).

Here are some exercises for opening your mind to the wonderful, expansive feeling it is possible to sustain in retreat.

> During the day when you are outside, open up your view to the horizon.
>
> Also open your view to the whole sky—notice the clouds and the sky behind them.
>
> Study the similarity between clouds and your thoughts; see how both come and go. This is opening to the open space in your mind—the "sky" in your mind.
>
> At night, open to the sky and stars. In retreat you have the unique opportunity to "star bathe". You can do this on a clear night by using a blanket to lie on your back on the ground so that your mind and body are completely open to the night sky.

Lifeflow retreats

The Lifeflow Centre runs a wide variety of retreats. Our public retreats are run over weekends or a whole week, and are guided by teachers who give theory classes and guide the meditation sessions. The teachers are also available for individual consultations for students who wish to discuss their experience. Plenty of time is set aside to enjoy the countryside where the retreat centre is located. The retreats are fully catered with beautiful food.

Each retreat takes a theme, which is explored during the retreat along with guided group meditations, yoga classes, deep relaxation, walks and time for individual meditation.

This chapter brings us to the close of Part One. Having explored what meditation is, how to develop calm and concentration, maintaining a healthy state of mind and moving from a point of balance, we are now going to explore the advanced material for Calm and Concentration: the deeper states of absorption and how you can further develop your meditation practice.

Part Two: Developing a meditation practice

Chapter 12: The levels of absorption– the transpersonal states

Each time you meditate, you start by noticing how busy your mind is, and then gradually settle into the meditation. Then you will naturally move up and down the levels of absorption.

In Chapter 5, I outlined in detail the three deepening stages of meditation. To refresh your memory, those three stages are:

1. You notice how busy your mind is as you see the thoughts rushing around. You are watching your thoughts instead of being driven by them.

2. Your thoughts slow down so that you can see them coming and going. You become aware of the spaces between the thoughts.

3. Your mind and emotions become so balanced that your thinking pauses for a while.

I also explained that in the second stage, when your thoughts slow down, you enter the first level of absorption. This absorbed state will deepen as you continue to meditate, and there are four levels of absorption you can begin to recognise. It is possible to develop the first level of absorption, and occasionally the second, in everyday life; the other levels can only be attained in formal meditation. This chapter explores how to recognise the levels of absorption, provides meditations to hold the different levels and describes the infinite absorptions.

The levels of absorption described in this chapter have been an integral part of the meditation tradition for thousands of years. Experienced meditators can recognise them clearly. However, no-one has previously discovered if the objective tests of neuroscience actually tally with what meditators have been describing.

The Lifeflow Meditation Centre was approached by a student at Flinders University to collaborate in an experiment to test these levels of absorption. Subsequently, thirteen Lifeflow Meditation students were wired up in the EEG unit of the University while they moved through these different levels. Experts in the fields of medicine, neuroscience, psychology, informatics and engineering were brought in to monitor the tests.

Even to the most sceptical, the results were clear cut. The measurements of brain wave activity confirmed the subjective experience described by the meditators. The experiment showed that participants entered a meditative state quickly at level 1, and that there was a clear progression through each level. The sleep specialists were fascinated to note that level 1 paralleled the process of going to sleep, except that the meditators stopped just before the point of sleep and then held this state between being asleep and awake[5]. The success of this experiment has led to a Ph.D. project with 20 Lifeflow Meditation students.

Level 1—Seeing the spaces between thoughts

The first level of absorption is the state you enter at the second deepening stage of meditation, and it contains the five qualities of an absorbed state:

- Your thinking is clear and effective
- Your emotions are calm
- Your body is relaxed
- Your mind is focused and
- You are in a state of physical, emotional and mental balance.

It can be recognised by a feeling of ease, with everything flowing smoothly. Thinking is still present but not disturbing; in fact, all productive thinking is done in this state.

In an absorbed state there is a sense of clarity, interest in what is happening, and joy, which can range from very subtle to utterly rapturous. Because your mind is focused completely on meditation it does not register any external sensory input, and the sounds and other disturbances which surround you can completely disappear.

For many years I taught meditation at The University of Adelaide and initially the only space available was near the cafeteria kitchens at lunchtime. Cooks were coming and going, pots and pans, plates, knives and forks were being washed and thrown around. Before moving into the main session I would always ask the class to meditate on all the sounds around them. After the meditation, everyone said that the sounds completely disappeared so they had meditated happily without the slightest disturbance.

Similarly, when people experiencing physical pain enter an absorbed state they find that pain moves into the background and may disappear while they are in that state. This is because the mind becomes so focused that, like the sounds in the kitchen, any disturbing input stops being registered. Meditation can thus be extremely valuable for managing chronic pain.

This state of absorption is what all athletes, sportspeople, artists, musicians, writers and scientists look for—it's where you "enter the zone" and what you are doing becomes effortless. Your mind and body work together in complete harmony, and this can deepen to the second level, where your thinking stops and you work by responding directly to what is happening, without having to think about it.

Level 2—Thinking stops

At the second level of absorption, your thinking stops. This happens naturally and Transcendental Meditation calls it *transcendence*. Your mind becomes so focused on the meditation object that it no longer needs to think about it. It simply rests there, in the sense experience of your body, quite still, not needing to wander off. At this stage a number of inner experiences might open up including **imagery, inner movements, joy, release of physical and emotional knots** and **deep peace**.

Imagery

You might experience washes of colour, points of light or incredibly clear visions—called *hypnagogic imagery*—as your mind opens up to experiences beyond your normal thought processes. At this stage, even if you are meditating on an external object, the object becomes completely internalised—it has been absorbed.

Inner movements

You might begin to feel yourself turning around, or rocking gently, as you tune in to the inner experiences of your body. You might also feel yourself suddenly sink, or start to float, but you will find that physically you have not moved; they are all inner experiences.

Joy

Because your mind is so still, a feeling of real joy arises; there is a feeling of union or connection with the meditation object because you are no longer thinking about it. At this level joy can expand into full ecstasy, one of the most pleasurable experiences possible, even greater than that of sex or orgasm.

Release of physical and emotional knots

When we first experience these levels of absorption it is often for a brief period, sometimes just a split second. Even so, the effect can be profound and last for up to three days. When your mind becomes so still that thinking actually stops, your mind and body are totally unified and this can have profound effects on your physical and mental health. Habitual physical and emotional knots dissolve, and there can be a sense of incredible release.

Deep peace

This is the depth of the mind—still and peaceful. Thoughts and emotions will pass by and not interfere at all; it is a place of deep inner peace.

At first it is difficult to recognise when you have reached the second level of absorption because you are not thinking. When you start thinking again and wonder what happened, or where you were (and so come out of the second absorption), you will recognise the state you were in. At this point you have returned to the first level of absorption or have moved out of the absorptions altogether. However, you will find it easy to maintain your calm and concentration.

Level 3—Body asleep, mind awake

At the third level of absorption your mind and body become so still that even the emotional reaction of joy stops. The mental state is very fine and you are left with a feeling of deep contentment, peace and happiness. Your body has reached the same stage as it does when it is asleep: deeply relaxed to the point where you can't move even if you want to (and you won't!). The difference between this state and sleep is that you are fully conscious, and your mind is clear, alert and concentrated. At this level you will experience **feelings of heaviness or lightness**, a sense of your **body boundaries dissolving**, and **no separation** between you and the meditation object.

Feelings of heaviness or lightness

As you move into this level of absorption and your body relaxes, it will feel very heavy. However, as this third level of absorption deepens, your body may begin to feel light.

Body boundaries dissolving

We all carry mental images of our bodies and the boundaries of our body and as these disappear we experience our bodies directly—

without any sense of boudaries at all. At this level of absorption, our sense of spatial orientation dissolves as our instinctive, automatic mental processes of referencing become still.

No separation

In the third level of absorption, the meditation object feels an integral part of your mind and your body and you feel no separation between your mind and body—they are completely unified. You are left with your direct physical sensations and you are actually in them—not separate from them. Because your body image and sense of spatial orientation have dissolved, you might feel as though you are floating in space, without any sense of direction.

Level 4—The breathing pauses

At the fourth level of absorption, you don't experience any physical sensations or feelings; it's as though your body has disappeared. The entire mind-body is so balanced that there is no movement whatsoever, physically, emotionally or mentally. There is a deep sense of stillness and concentration, which is alive and deeply satisfying.

In this deeply balanced state the breathing can pause, and this is how you can recognise this level of absorption. Like becoming aware of thinking when it begins again, you will become aware that the breathing has paused when it naturally begins again.

During the process of absorption, the breathing becomes increasingly slow and fine, so when it does pause it is hardly noticeable at first. You breathe out, and there will be a brief pause before breathing in again. As the ability to hold an absorbed state develops, it can last for a much longer time.

Moving up and down the levels

Each time you meditate, you will start by noticing how busy your mind is, and then gradually settle into the meditation. Then you will naturally move up and down the levels of absorption.

Usually you will experience the first level of absorption every time you formally meditate. (You may also touch this level each time you do a Spot Meditation.) The other levels you will touch briefly as you meditate, often only for a split second. This is normal, because it is only through practice that you will hold them for a longer period of time (see the chart over the page which describes how to do this).

As you develop a practice and begin to recognise the levels of absorption, you can hold them by gently letting go of your thoughts and bringing your focus back to the meditation object. It feels like you are allowing yourself to sink back into the sea—just floating.

Recognising which level of absorption you are in

The following chart summarises the qualities of each level of absorption, to help you recognise them.

Level of absorption	Qualities of the absorption
1st absorption	Body relaxed. Mind calm. Mind focused on single object or task, eg counting. or breathing, without wandering. Thinking is still present, but all thoughts and images are directed to same goal.
2nd absorption	Thinking stops. Inner movements and experiences may open up. Still have a sense of body boundaries. Deeper connection with feelings and sensations in body and a sense of joy.
3rd absorption	Body becomes very heavy, can't move, sense of having sunk. No emotion. Body boundaries dissolve, just have sensation. Breathing still regular.
4th absorption	Breathing slows to almost nothing and will pause. No sensations or feelings—very still.

Meditations to hold the different levels of absorption

The chart below describes how you can use different breathing meditations to hold each level of absorption.

Level of absorption	Meditation to use
1st absorption	*Watching the breath* and counting from 1 to 60. Repeat as long as you wish. Keep your mind focused on counting. Count as follows: in-breath, out-breath, 1; in-breath, out-breath, 2; etc. Alternatively, count your pulse (heart beat) or just count seconds. Remember to keep the counting going—don't let yourself drift into a deeper state.
2nd absorption	*Wave Breath* • Feel the in and out breath move through your torso, gently massaging it. • Expand the out-breath through your body. Or imagine the breath moving up and down your body as you breathe in and out. • Notice the sensations through your body.

Level of absorption	Meditation to use
3rd absorption	*Nourishing Breath* Slightly slow down the in-breath and focus the breath into the heart centre (or navel centre). Let body boundaries dissolve, allow feeling of heaviness and/or sinking. Keep your breathing going, don't let it drop to almost nothing.
4th absorption	*Nourishing Breath* Focus on the out-breath—"breathing out to the end of the breath" Let the out-breath slow down. Let the breath naturally pause and rest in the space at the end of the breath.

The fourth level of absorption is the deepest level attainable and at this level you can continue down the path of absorptions—to the infinite absorptions—or use this state to develop insight.

The infinite absorptions

If you continue down the path of absorptions, there are four more levels called the *infinite absorptions*, which are actually developments of the fourth level of absorption. The mind doesn't go any deeper, but the concentration is so fine and the mind so inner-directed, that it moves away from the meditation object and focuses on inner experiences. These levels of absorption are the basis for all mystical experiences across different cultures and religions, and they go beyond any boundaries we set.

Level 5—Infinite space
At level 5, the mind opens up to the experience of *infinite space*. There is no defined object in the mind because it has gone beyond anything that has a shape or form, to penetrate to the matrix of everything that exists, which is space. The mind opens up completely, without limits, boundaries or perspective, to an infinite vista. One image to describe this is a horizon-less sky.

(A note of caution: this experience is not necessarily a physical reality, but a concept the mind is capable of experiencing.)

Level 6—Infinite consciousness
At this level of absorption, you experience a shift in perception; it's as though the experience of infinite space becomes vibrant. This is the absorption of *infinite consciousness*, and it is the experience of consciousness as infinite. Although we can accept the concept of

space being infinite, we are not so comfortable with the concept of *consciousness* being infinite.

This experience raises the possibility of a level of consciousness beyond the normal boundaries we ascribe to it. When we speak of something being conscious we usually mean that it is *self*-conscious. Experiencing the sixth level of absorption reveals that there is the possibility of a level of consciousness beyond all forms and boundaries and therefore beyond self-consciousness. It suggests that self-consciousness is only one form of consciousness; or to put it another way, self-consciousness is a *product* of consciousness.

The 13th century church scholar and mystic, Meister Eckhart, said there was something beyond God, which he called the *Godhead*[6]. It is probable that he opened up to this experience of infinite consciousness because he was attempting to describe something beyond any known form or concept.

In Western philosophy and psychology we assume that consciousness is a by-product of complex development. However, in meditation you can experience *consciousness itself*. In a sense, consciousness becomes its own object.

The Insight stream of meditation explores this question thoroughly. Insight meditation goes beyond concepts to direct experience, so it can take you beyond the concept of infinite consciousness to the experience of a fundamental level of consciousness without any sense of self. There is no self-referencing at all so you do not experience something else as an object separate from yourself. There is no "you", there is no object, there is only consciousness.

I like to make a clear distinction between fundamental consciousness and self-consciousness by using the term *awareness* for fundamental consciousness. Awareness is an in-built ability to respond to stimulus. Every atom is aware, in the sense that it forms ordered relationships. Insight meditation reveals that awareness is a property of the universe, like matter and energy, and from this fundamental property all of the qualities we understand as consciousness arise[7]. So the sixth level of absorption is a prelude to the experience of fundamental awareness. However, the absorptions do not stop at this point.

Level 7—Nothingness

The next level is called the *sphere of nothingness*. Even subtle objects or concepts like infinite consciousness dissolve and what is left can only be described as nothingness. However, it can be experienced. It's like resting in a void but there is still a sense of perceiving "something" even though it is nothingness, a bit like deep space, without any light, or like dropping into a velvety, all-embracing darkness.

Level 8—The boundary of perception

At this level of absorption, we reach the *boundaries of perception* and cannot say whether anything is being perceived or not. It is called "neither perception nor non-perception" in the meditation tradition. We have also gone beyond the boundaries of Western logic, because at this level something cannot be said to exist or not exist—the distinction between the mind and any kind of object has completely dissolved.

Usually these last four levels of absorption can only be experienced under retreat conditions, and at Level 8 your mind is as still and fine as possible, so this is the end of the line.

I have outlined the infinite levels of absorption for three reasons. The first is that someone who has developed a meditation practice might drop into these states and wonder what happened. The second is that these experiences open up philosophical questions and answers our culture is battling with, and here are concrete, demonstrable and testable experiences which open the mind to states of consciousness way beyond our normal understanding. Finally, these experiences clarify that the mind is actually infinite, in the sense that it can expand beyond any boundaries.

Dropping into nothingness

The first time I experienced going beyond the level of *infinite consciousness* was during a year-long retreat in Assisi. The members of the household decided to meet one evening, and before the meeting I sat down to meditate. After an hour I emerged from the meditation and went to the living room for the meeting, but no-one was there. I went back and checked my watch and found that instead of my normal hour's meditation I had been meditating for well over two hours. The meeting was long finished.

I knew I hadn't been asleep, but I had no concept of time having passed at all—it was as though I had dropped into deep, velvety space: a complete void. I had recognised the experiences of infinite space and consciousness, but after that—nothing. I lost all sense of time, space and everything else.

Years later a student came to see me very disturbed, because he had dropped into the same experience. He was extremely relieved to find I could explain it to him.

The myth of unconsciousness

The infinite absorptions have been an integral part of the meditation tradition for 3000 years, and they open up a view of consciousness which goes beyond self-consciousness. They also take the mind to the limits of our perception.

The experience of infinite consciousness throws into question the whole notion of *unconsciousness*. As discussed earlier, in the West consciousness refers to self-consciousness, and from this point of view there is a state of unconsciousness. However, if there is a level of consciousness *beyond* self-consciousness, then at this more fundamental level *awareness* is a given, and unconsciousness is the shadow cast by the limited view of self-consciousness—it is simply a by-product of self-consciousness.

In other words, our senses are receptive to stimuli all the time—they are always aware. Through developing our thinking and sense of self, we learn to ignore most of this information most of the time. It's there, but it's in the shadow, outside the realm of our self-consciousness.

The human mind is infinite

Experiencing the infinite absorptions also clarifies that the mind is actually infinite in the sense that it can expand beyond any boundaries.

Human beings repeatedly try to expand their physical existence. We collect things, attempting to own more and more, we colonise, we build up our bodies, and we seem to believe that it's possible to develop our economy infinitely—that it must always be in a state of growth.

Even a casual observation of nature reveals that nothing grows infinitely. Every form of life is limited by its ability to sustain itself and the conditions that support it. As a culture we are horrified by decay so completely ignore it. We want to grow infinitely and the danger is that we confuse cancerous growth with development.

I think we feel that *something* is infinite, and much suffering is caused by trying to fulfill this physically. If our culture became aware that consciousness and therefore our minds are actually infinite, it might be easier to distinguish between this feeling of infinity, between the nature of our minds and the reality of our bodies, and perhaps be more accepting of the finite, limited nature of our bodies.

As mentioned earlier, the fourth level of absorption can also be used to develop insight.

Developing insight

As the fourth level of absorption is the deepest level attainable, where the mind-body is completely balanced, it is the optimum state for seeing directly and clearly. There are no disturbances whatsoever, and the mind is completely focused. Instead of turning in and moving to the infinite levels of absorption, you can use this state to develop insight and wisdom. This is done by moving from a receptive, open state of mind, to sharpening the focus and developing a penetrative quality of mind.

It can be described as a state of question. Because the mind has become extremely still, raising a question will disturb it, but not enough to knock it out of balance. It takes the mind out of this deeply absorbed state very slightly, so that we are aware both externally and internally. We have accessed our self-referencing consciousness while being deeply absorbed. (This can happen spontaneously, especially if, as in Zen, the state of question has been developed from the start by the use of *koans*, for example.) This is how we open to our intuition––instead of trying to discover something through thinking or feelings, we have access to the whole mind-body and will *see directly into the question*. We will be the question and in being the question, *experience the answer* completely as the entire mind-body responds. (Refer to my book *Insight and Love* for further information.)

The steps for developing insight are quite different from those used to develop the absorptions. This is why different schools of meditation contradict each other. Zen, for example, focuses totally on developing insight, so its preliminary instructions demand alertness at the cost of relaxation. However, I prefer to teach in a way that covers all the different streams of the tradition, because it provides the tools and techniques to lead a fulfilling and balanced life.

The next chapter discusses what happens when we don't achieve the calm and concentrated state of the absorptions. It examines emotions in more detail and describes how you can use meditation to work with them more skillfully.

Chapter 13: Working with emotions

The meditation tradition understands how emotions work and provides the tools and techniques to work with them.

It's comforting to know that unhealthy states of mind have always been accepted as an integral part of meditation, and come in the training package with their own list! We can lose the plot, get caught in emotional turmoil, seethe with rage, become consumed by lust or jealousy, give way to arrogance or fall apart at the seams and completely run out of energy. The first major hurdle is simply accepting that the human mind does this and that we all get dumped in the waves of emotions at different times.

Let's return to the analogy of the sea—on a calm day it can be totally still and clear. This is what the mind is like when it is absorbed. With some wind around, the sea begins to whip up and form waves and these can build into huge breakers. This can be exhilarating if you are watching safely, but if you are actually in the sea it's another story altogether. When the mind gets whipped up, it can literally seethe and boil, just like the sea in a storm. (Have you seen old movies where sex scenes are very discreet? As the passion builds and the lovers move towards each other to kiss, the camera inevitably pans to an image of the sea—the waves crash against rocks and the music soars.)Welcome to the world of emotions.

When we stand on a wild beach we know how to protect ourselves. We know we are dealing with enormously powerful forces and we respect them. If we are not interested, or don't have the resources, we don't engage with them. But if we do want to ride the waves, sail, or camp on a wild beach, we take it seriously and make sure we have the appropriate equipment.

Emotions are exactly the same as these powerful natural forces. However, as we are left to deal with emotions without any training, we don't really understand the forces we are dealing with. The meditation tradition understands how emotions work and provides the tools and techniques to work with them.

Respecting the natural power of emotions

If we view emotions as powerful, natural forces, we can bring to them the same respect we would to any other force in nature. This is the best protection we have against getting caught in them. Respecting our emotions will free us from being either completely blind to them or afraid of them, which usually leads to denying their existence or repression. These were often the only options available as we grew, but since Freud people have understood that denied and repressed emotions will surface sooner or later and, because we are not looking, catch us unawares.

By respecting them we can come to know them and recognise the conditions that bring them about. We can see overwhelming waves coming, and dive under them or ensure we stay on the beach when they are around.

Meditation is the best way to learn about emotional forces because it provides a genuine alternative to denial or repression. By providing the means to step back and just watch, meditation creates the space in which we can accept and come to know our emotions and how they work.

Acceptance, wanting and dissatisfaction

Acceptance, then, is the first step. If we don't accept that something exists we can't see it, so have no way of understanding it. The Rolling Stones expressed the essence of Buddhist philosophy in two of their songs, *You Can't Always Get What You Want* and *I Can't Get No Satisfaction*[8]. When Mick Jagger wails, yells and struts these lyrics he is expressing the two fundamental drives that stir the mind into a storm: wanting and dissatisfaction.

Wanting is insatiable, because it has nothing to do with the reality of our bodies. Stuck in our minds, we find that when we get what we want, the bottom line changes. Enough is never satisfying, and when enough is not enough, more is never enough! Because we are ignoring the reality of our senses—not taking the time to feel and register what our bodies are actually experiencing—we remain dissatisfied. Instead of a million dollars being plenty; as someone once told me, "A million dollars is nothing nowadays!"

Wanting and dissatisfaction are completely intertwined, and from them arises the whole repertoire of emotional upheaval. So when we get caught in waves and lose the calm and concentration of the absorptions, we can be sure these emotions are at the root of whatever we are experiencing.

The song *You Can't Always Get What You Want* continues with *But if you try sometimes, well you just might find, you get what you need*—and this is the key. Without desire we wouldn't be able to live: a healthy desire to live is essential for survival. There are also needs which have to be fulfilled; and then we like to play because in playing we learn. So the human race has built culture, which means that our desire to learn, play and lead a happy and fulfilling life (instead of just surviving) is possible.

However, like everything in life there is a balance point, and when our desires become obsessive and lose touch with the reality of our needs, we start to experience the emotional knots and blocks which form the seeds of emotional storms.

Getting caught in the waves of emotions

When we get caught in emotional waves, the mind closes in on itself—instead of being grounded in the body and senses, thoughts feed off each other, causing a closed loop. The mind becomes stuck, and "stuckness" is the basic ingredient of wanting. We are driven by its force, unable to see beyond the turbulence created by our minds, swirling faster and faster as our thoughts spin out of control.

I have called it *wanting* but there are a constellation of emotions that give a sense of this feeling: craving, yearning, possessiveness and greed are some of them. At the core is a feeling of self-pity, a sense of missing out, and this is exactly what is happening because, being stuck in a closed circuit of thought, we have completely lost touch with the immediate experience of our bodies. We are missing out on the experience of our senses. This comes through wanting life to be somehow different from how it actually is.

In an absorbed state, the mind-body is connected and balanced. The mind is steadily focused on a single object and impressions from the senses flow smoothly through it. We are connected with life and our senses are open to what is around us, so we feel whole and integrated. When the mind becomes stuck in thoughts about what is happening, has happened, or could happen, it splits off from the body and begins to churn like a breaking wave. The idea takes over from reality and when this happens the mind is stuck in wanting. We create an unhealthy state of mind that blocks us from seeing clearly and cuts us off from our surroundings.

Acceptance is the first step in dealing with this unhealthy state because even if we have good reason for wanting to change something about our lives, we can't do it if we don't accept where we actually are and see clearly the situation we are in. It's like trying to apply a cure to a disease without even making a diagnosis.

The stages of the wave

When we want something different from what is actually happening, there are five stages in the wave of emotion that arises: **wanting, dissatisfaction, confusion and denial, worry and anxiety** and eventually **loss of confidence**. This wave has been described in detail in the meditation tradition and I think it summarises neatly the common psychological disorders. It explains what happens when the mind gets into an unhealthy state and you will find, as you become familiar with the five stages, that they always follow the same course.

Wanting

Every time you run into trouble in meditation or life, your mind has started wanting something: wanting a particular result, wanting to repeat the good experience that happened yesterday, wanting to get rid of the headache, wanting to buy a new car, wanting your partner to understand, wanting to change what happened at work, wanting to feel good, wanting the neighbours to shut up, wanting a cup of coffee—and so on. It's endless. When this begins you have become caught in a wave. As the wave rolls on you will find that, like all waves, it follows a particular pattern.

Dissatisfaction

Wanting is inevitably followed by dissatisfaction. When we don't get what we want, the mind starts to reject the whole idea of wanting it anyway. If you observe a young child you will see this clearly: "If I can't have it, then I don't want it anyway!" Even if we do get what we want, we eventually become dissatisfied with it. So we reject what is happening by becoming angry, bored, critical and judgmental or even afraid.

Confusion and denial

The wave rolls on and the third stage is a state of confusion, exactly like being tossed in a wave and having no idea what is up, down, forwards or backwards. Having become caught in wanting and then dissatisfaction, we run out of energy and can't even be clear about what we wanted in the first place. We end up denying that we wanted anything at all and can't be bothered any more. We don't care. Sleepiness sets in: we feel lethargic and sluggish and don't want to do anything. However, the wave doesn't stop at this point.

Worry and anxiety

At this stage, we find that whether we wanted, didn't want or didn't care doesn't make any difference—we are caught, so we begin to panic and become anxious. The mind gives up any illusion of being in control of the situation and realises that the wave is going to continue no matter what is done. Any sense of direction has gone and, not seeing any way out, we become stressed.

Loss of confidence

Finally the wave breaks and we are left feeling wrung out. Our confidence has been shattered by becoming caught in something we had absolutely no control over, and we doubt our abilities. Left dumped on the beach, we wonder if anything is worth it at all. Chucking it all in appears to be the only option as everything seems too hard. Decisions are impossible and depression can loom on the horizon. The mind, having completely lost its connection with the body, and therefore an anchor to hold it still or a rudder to steer it, has become shipwrecked. This is the end of the line.

To summarise, the stages the mind goes through once it is caught in a wave are:

1. Wanting something else to happen
2. Becoming dissatisfied, angry and bored
3. Denying that we wanted anything and becoming lethargic and sluggish
4. Becoming stressed, anxious and worried
5. Losing confidence and feeling worthless

Coming out of the wave

When we become angry or dissatisfied it means we wanted something. When depression, anxiety and worthlessness take hold it means we don't even know what we wanted any more. The simplest way to recover from this is just to be honest and admit that we wanted something. Though the concept is simple, it's not always easy, because often there is pain and perhaps humiliation in admitting to ourselves that what we wanted didn't happen.

The bulk of clinical psychological work is structured around developing a healthy, functioning identity, so it is basically centred on the self. The knowledge and strategies developed for helping this process are invaluable and, although meditation can be a valuable tool in this process, it cannot be a substitute for these. Meditation opens up a completely different perspective—one that goes beyond the self––and this is why the two disciplines complement each other so well. Let's revisit the wave of emotion, comparing the two perspectives.

From the self's point of view the outcome of the wave is catastrophic. All appears to be lost; control and direction have gone and decision making seems impossible. Life has lost its meaning. Because we see the self as permanent and stable, by the time we are dumped by the wave we believe that this is a permanent situation. There seems to be no way out—and *from the self's point of view* this has a certain amount of truth in it.

However, let's look at it another way. If you have ever been caught in a wave, you know that eventually it breaks on the beach, and you are washed ashore. From the *point of view of meditation*, this is exactly what has happened. Anger, lethargy, anxiety, worthlessness and meaninglessness are not the bottom line—the beach is. This is the balanced, still, and spacious foundation of our minds; the state where our minds and bodies are balanced.

In meditation you discover that all waves of emotion come and go; no state of mind is permanent. Beyond every healthy and unhealthy state of mind, is the still, spacious quality of the foundation of consciousness. All states of mind depend on this foundation for their existence, and will always settle back into it and return to a state of balance.

When the mind becomes disturbed, all we need to do is sit still and the disturbance will pass. Like a wave, it will eventually break and wash onto the beach. Experiencing this brings enormous confidence, because it provides a broader perspective: knowing that disturbing emotions are not the whole picture. They exist within a vast ocean of consciousness, the nature of which is open, spacious and still.

What this means is that the foundation of our minds, and of our nature, is not despair like the existentialists believed, or original sin, or even hope or fear. It is the depth of consciousness—that state of deep, still balance—that we can experience through meditation. Knowing this and being able to contact it whenever we choose, we can immediately step out of any disturbing emotional state, and get back to the beach. We can move at will from an unhealthy state of mind to a healthy, absorbed state of mind.

Learning the patterns of the mind

As you come to know your mind better, you will become accustomed to its changing states and not worry so much about them. The human mind is a product of nature, and it functions according to the same laws. Waking and going to sleep are the sunrise and sunset of our minds, clouds come and go as we feel bright or dull, and wind can churn up our emotional waves. This is simply the way our mind works and we cannot directly control it. However, we can observe how it works and begin to understand the conditions that create certain states, and the laws under which it operates.

The more we understand these laws, the more able we are to work with them, because we can see things coming instead of them catching us unawares. We know where the beach is, which conditions create a calm state, how storms arise, see waves coming and know which ones to ride or how to get out of the way, where it is shallow and where it is deep.

Perfection and The Three "Musterbations"

One major reason for not seeing how the mind works, or even accepting it, is the illusion of perfection. This catches nearly all of us and I am indebted to the American psychologist Albert Ellis for his summary of the three obsessions that create this illusion[8]. He calls them *The Three Musterbations:*

1. I must be well all the time and everything I do must be the best.

2. Everyone else must do what I want, treat me well and those who are important to me must love me.

3. The economy and the environment I live in must work for me. (That is, the world around me must be organised to suit me.)

This is wanting taken to the extreme of musterbating. It is impossible for anyone to be the best all the time and we have no control over other people, so expecting them to do what we want and to always like us, is absurd. And of course neither the economy nor the environment we live in is focused on us.

Trying to make life fit into a preordained set of "musts" makes it impossible to see how our minds actually work, because we can't accept whatever happens. We need to be able to accept what happens, without wishing that it were different, to see clearly what is happening and give ourselves a chance to work with life and the people with whom we share it.

When we want something to be perfect we usually mean that we want it to conform to our idea of how it should be. If we look at perfection in this sense, life is not, and never could be perfect. If our minds are obsessed with "musts" and aiming for perfection, the body can't get a look-in because it is only capable of being *real*. So our mind splits off from the body and this means the mind is going in one direction, the body in another, and our emotions are caught in a state of conflict. However, perfect actually means "complete", and being *complete* in the sense of keeping the mind, emotions and body connected is not an impossible aim.

When we are absorbed there is no conflict: the mind is supported by the body and therefore the two are *completely* united. Our senses are open and we are in touch with what is actually happening—we can see things as they really are. So we know what the mind is experiencing at any particular time and we can adjust accordingly. We can see any wave that comes and don't have to become caught in it. In other words, we know exactly where we are internally and externally.

When you are caught in a wave it means that you didn't see it coming. If you do become caught, your mind was probably occupied with one of The Three Musterbations. They take you straight out of the absorptions into the emotional turmoil of wanting and dissatisfaction.

For example, while meditating you might be thinking about something that happened during the day: your shoulder feels sore, you are annoyed about the mechanic not fixing the car, you can't have that wonderful feeling you had in meditation yesterday and your mind won't stay still. Every time you meditate it should be peaceful and feel good, otherwise it is a waste of time—and you start to worry about the meditation not being up to its usual standard. As soon as the worrying begins, you move out of an absorbed state and are caught by a wave.

By expecting that meditation should always go well and be free from thoughts and bits and pieces of daily life, the mind starts musterbating. It loses its anchor in the body and is swept into a closed circle of thinking that has nothing to do with what is actually happening. The body doesn't stop experiencing—it can't, because the senses keep operating—so the mind and body are no longer whole in the sense that they are not connected or working together.

The moment you bring your mind back and accept what your body is actually experiencing, the worrying stops and you come back to an absorbed state. Even if you are thinking, have a headache and are annoyed, if you are noticing this and not expecting something else to be happening, you are in a calm and concentrated state and your meditation is going well.

Becoming friends with yourself

It's odd that we are so intolerant of ourselves, feeling that our bodies need to be controlled, to stop them going berserk. We are the only person we have to live with for the whole of our lives and we are usually taught not to trust ourselves or our bodies.

As we begin to build a meditation practice, this lack of trust comes increasingly to the foreground, because the feeling that our bodies should do exactly what we want when we want it, is based on the assumption that our minds are separate from our bodies.

Our philosophical tradition assumes that the body is a soft machine which the mind drives. This automatically creates a feeling that our bodies are alien from who we really are, so we find it extremely difficult to experience our bodies on their own terms, or to trust them. Under these conditions it is virtually impossible to feel safe in our bodies and many people spend their lives trying to get out of their bodies or attempting to live as though their bodies don't exist.

This is a real shame, because without our bodies we have no life. The reason for training yourself to accept what is happening *without trying to change it* is to become aware of your body on its own terms—as a living, conscious organism—instead of trying to force it to conform to an image.

If your body were a machine it wouldn't feel anything and yet the direct experience of your body is feeling. This is the only way the body can be experienced. Imagine how much of our lives are cut out because we don't want to feel what is happening, or can't feel it. With our minds and bodies alienated, is it any wonder we don't feel comfortable much of the time? We hope that if we gain approval from others we will feel better, yet everything we feel comes from our own minds and bodies, not from anyone else.

Through meditating we can accept, come to know, and become friends with ourselves. This is the ground on which a happy life can grow, in which you can become friends with others, and in which you can open up to the true being of your body as an integral part of life, earth and the universe.

The next chapter discusses how to make decisions using the **Three C Technique**.

Chapter 14: Making decisions using the Three C Technique

The Three C Technique can be used long before a wave arises to determine whether we will catch it or not.

Making decisions is very much like surfing. If your mind is turbulent it's best to either stay on the beach or just dive under the turbulence––there's no point trying to make any decision in this state. However, we have all run into the feeling that we should do something about the turbulence, and that's often when we try to make a decision. It's fatal! And it always will be, because we are moving from an unbalanced state.

Decision making is a function of the mind, and it's a process you can learn about and join in or you can attempt to ignore, but you can't stop it from happening. In fact, experiments have discovered that often a decision is made in the brain before we become aware of it[10]. So trying to stop or ignore the process is rather like trying to stop or ignore waves on the sea. It's much more fulfilling and fun to learn how to ride these movements of the mind.

This chapter explores how the Three C Technique can be used to make decisions.

What is a decision?

The word *decide* has its root in the Latin *decidere* which brings together two words *de*, meaning "away", and *caedere*, "to cut". So the act of decision has its root meaning in cutting something way, and a decision does mean choosing one option among many—cutting that option away from the infinite possibilities we face. Instead of the way ahead being open and full of potential, it becomes limited and bound to follow a certain direction. However, to move it is necessary to do this.

There are three typical ways we tend to make decisions:

1. The first is that we can't bear having to think about something––we'd rather just get on with it.

This is the entrepreneur who trusts his or her gut feeling and runs with that, having very little patience for someone who is more cautious and wants to check out the situation carefully.

2. The second tends to procrastination because we feel we need to think about ever more information before being able to decide.

An academic tends to follow this way, trusting his or her thinking above all and wanting to discuss and weigh things up for ever, often becoming paralysed in the process.

3. The third leads to feeling overwhelmed because we can see all the options and know that if we choose one we will have to miss out on the others.

A shop owner told me that when he only had one or two flavours of ice-cream life was much simpler. Now, with over ten different flavours, children would stand for ages in front of them not being able to make up their minds, while the shop filled with other children impatiently waiting their turn.

This is the nature of decisions: "If I catch this wave there might be a better one coming, or it might end up dumping me anyway". Once we catch the wave we are on our way. Remembering that a decision can only ever be a work in progress because there is no final solution; letting go of trying to always get things right; realising that all waves come and go and being prepared to learn, all make the process much easier.

Trying to avoid making decisions is impossible, because we have to move to live. The only choice we really have is whether we make decisions consciously or unconsciously.

Research on good decision making

A recent article outlined findings on how to make good decisions based on research conducted with students at the University of Amsterdam[11]. With very simple decisions students did better when they thought about it, but when it came to more complex decisions they did much better *not* thinking about it.

The team conducting the research proposed that our brains subconsciously churn through a mass of information, sifting out the best options. Psychologist Daniel Kahneman at Princeton University notes that many complicated processes occur without our being aware of it. He suggests sleeping on a big decision to allow the intuition to come into play.

Our culture has no method to train intuition. Unlike thinking it is left to chance—you either sleep on something or follow a feeling, without having much idea of how it works or how to check it. The Three C Technique is a way to use your intuition with precision whenever you choose. You don't have to leave anything to chance and can access both parts of your brain—thinking *and* the subconscious, your mind *and* body—through checking out the options, forming the question clearly, and then meditating on it.

The Three C Technique applied to decision making

One of the great advantages of applying the Three C Technique to making decisions is that you can establish your mental balance before taking action. You can be aware of what is happening right at the moment the action begins—and all actions begin in our minds. Being faced with a decision is the moment we become conscious of this, because we know that what we decide will determine what happens in our lives for some time into the future, so it can be a very daunting process.

Catching the moment—asking the question

The first stage of making a decision is based on opening and becoming receptive to what you want or need to do. This is the step of **Catching the moment**, of becoming *aware* of where you are and what is happening and bringing the question in your mind out into the open, where you can focus on it.

The trickiest part is often formulating the question clearly—making it as simple and straightforward as possible. Once your question is clear, the answer is usually a simple *Yes* or *No*. If not, it is generally a sign that you are not really clear yet about the question you are asking.

When your question is clear, you use your thinking to collect information and look at the options. It is more active than just watching—you do whatever research you think is necessary. There are many strategies that can be adopted, such as making lists to weigh the pros and cons. Your personal research might also involve asking friends and advisers for their opinions and what they can see in the situation that you can't see.

Normally we would then act on our thinking and the advice given to us without going any further. But this only involves *half* of our minds and is the reason why many of our decisions have such strange and unpredictable outcomes. So the next step is to **Clear the space**.

Clearing the space

Stage one focused on formulating the question clearly; stage two is exactly the opposite—when you **Clear the space**, you also let go of the question. Moving to stage two of the decision-making process seems irrational, and it is. Our rational, conscious mind has done its work and we are now opening the other part of our mind—the non-rational, subconscious mind.

Clearing the space involves placing the question in your mind, then moving to a meditation exercise and letting go—giving up thinking about it altogether and allowing your mind to become as still as possible.

When your mind becomes still and absorbed, your mind and body are united and your mind is completely open to all the information stored in your body. Everything the body has experienced, everything stored in the memory and everything that is part of the body's history is open to the mind.

In this state we are open to our intuition, because intuition is this ability to be aware of the whole picture. For making a decision, you only need to balance the mind and body for a short time. Meditating formally for ten minutes or so, or even doing a Spot Meditation, brings the body into awareness.

By letting go of thinking about your question you allow your mind and body to respond, not from a particular point of view as the conscious mind does, but without any point of view at all. They respond from the whole of their experience. Your mind will make associations that would never occur to you if you tried to think about them, and this association process is fundamental to the intuition. Like a still, clear lake everything is reflected in your mind.

While meditating you will find that hopes and fears associated with the question will bubble up and it's best to let them come through, rather than trying to repress them and do the *right thing*. Just watch them in the same way you would notice any thoughts or emotions in meditation. Acknowledge everything you feel about deciding *Yes* or *No*. This will take the heat out of the decision.

Changing the habit—making the decision

Using your meditation as the anchor point, you will become increasingly balanced as your mind and body connect and you open to what your body is actually feeling. You can then take into account both what you have worked out with your thinking and what your body has registered through the senses. Your thinking and feeling can work together.

The third stage of making a decision using the Three C Technique is to register the response. There are three distinct ways to pick up the response of our minds and bodies. Some people find this easier to do than others, but with practice most people who are interested in meditating can get a feeling for this.

Types of responses

In Chapter 3 I noted that we all process information differently so let's quickly revise the three different ways people register things internally.

1. Some people see things in pictures, they **see** images and see what something means.
2. Some people have an internal conversation so will **hear** an answer.
3. Others base their actions on their feel for a situation. They will **feel** in their bodies what to do.

The response we receive depends on which sense we rely on to orient ourselves.

Visual response

Those people who think in pictures will find that their mind and body responds to their question through some kind of image. For example, one client asked whether she needed to leave her job. When she used the Three C Technique, a clear image of a dead fish arose in her mind, which really surprised her. However, there was no difficulty interpreting it and no need for any input from me. She left her job and has never looked back.

Aural response

For more aurally-oriented people the response can arise as a word. Again, this can be very direct and straightforward. For example, a client was very concerned about whether he needed to put in the enormous amount of work it would take to apply for a certain position in the company he worked for. The shock he received from his response was palpable because, as he said, "It can't possibly be that quick!" The answer was one direct word: "No".

So he put it to the test, went through with the application and interview and found that it would have been much more profitable to save his energy. The department offering the position was dissolved and the manager running the application process moved on. He now takes this process very seriously.

Feeling response

The third way to register a response is kinaesthetic, that is, through a direct feeling in the body. This can arise in a number of ways but is based on a feeling of balance right through the body as it settles into a response. The feeling can be centred in either the heart region or the abdomen; a "gut feeling" is the typical way this is described. There is a sense of the whole body being involved, of no division.

> As a professional musician working with contemporary music, I always knew immediately whether a piece of music was good. My confidence in this judgment came from my immediate physical response and it was only after learning meditation that I realised what I was doing. If a piece sent a shiver through my body and I could feel the hairs stand up around the back of my neck, I knew it was a good piece. This response stood the test of time repeatedly as composers I judged good gradually came into the public domain, and others were left behind. I never told anyone how I knew and people were perplexed at my confidence and track record, but it was as direct and simple as that.

Combining a feeling with visual or aural response

Sometimes a mixture of a kinaesthetic response and a word or vision can occur. So a vision, word, or even a sentence will arise along with a feeling of balance and "rightness" in the body.

Acting on the decision

After registering the response of the mind and body, the next step is to act on it. Naturally we have a goal in mind and a decision will have been made to move in that direction. However, while the mind is focused on an *idea* of where it wants to go—the goal—it is the *body* that actually has to go there, and this can only happen as it moves and adapts according to the circumstances and conditions of the living, changing situation it is in.

By allowing the mind to become balanced and still in the second stage of making the decision, the feelings and emotions associated with the decision that we cannot access with our conscious mind have been included in the process—the body has been taken into account. This enables us to focus on what is actually happening as we live through a decision, seeing each stage as it unfolds, rather than having a fixed view of what the outcome should be.

A fixed view comes from not taking account of the body. While the mind is fixated on a particular outcome, the changing circumstances of the situation will not be seen so we can be driven into a completely different direction from the one we set out on, much to our surprise. We find that we have simply reverted to well-trodden paths—the mind has trundled down the path of least resistance and old habits have reasserted themselves. The unconscious decisions of habit proved to be much stronger than the decision we thought we made.

The calm and stillness of meditation is the best possible basis on which to ground a decision because this calm, open state enables you to *stay aware as you act on the decision*. You have the chance to see clearly the link between the original decision and the results of the action. Seeing this link is the key to successful decision making, so that if, for example, your decision affected other people, or the environment around you in a way you couldn't have originally imagined, this can then be taken into account.

Another way to put this is to look at it from the perspective of the body. Some of us make decisions from our heads, through thinking about it. Others make them from their gut feelings. In the balanced state of meditation these two seemingly opposite and irreconcilable positions are brought together, and the mid-point between the head and the gut is the heart. This is the balance point of the mind-body, so a decision which is grounded here takes account of the habits of the body as well as the ideas of the mind.

Sometimes the decision you reach using the Three C Technique doesn't fit your expectations—only by acting on it will you see the results and discover whether it is a good one or not. You will then see whether your expectations were correct and whether you saw the situation clearly or not. If you weren't seeing it clearly, you now know and can quickly adjust your decision accordingly.

Decisions and values

Although we are not aware of it most of the time, the kinds of decisions we make are based on our values—the things which are important to us, what motivates us and what we see to be true. We might value success or honesty, status or friendship for example.

Sometimes these values live together rather uneasily and this can make more important decisions difficult. For example, you might have to face the option of lying for a friend, or the choice between taking a higher profile position which is more boring and an exciting job which pays less.

Different parts of us also have different value systems. For example, when at home we behave and treat people completely differently from when at work. Often these different parts with their different values are completely unknown to each other. So the more a decision affects our lives, the more these different value systems apply and the greater chance there is for conflict. This can produce considerable anxiety as we have to face our battle between security and challenge, or between following our passion and remaining within the comfort of our peer group for example.

One of the major advantages of using the Three C Technique for making decisions is that you have the space to detect the congruence or incongruence of your internal value systems. It will arise as you allow the feelings, images and thoughts associated with the question to come through while Clearing the space.

When still and balanced you can accept incongruent signals, and they can be included in the decision instead of being ignored. This can save an enormous amount of trouble, time and money when you act on your decision, because instead of being caught in the conflict of your ideas about what should be done, you are able to listen to your body. *Your body is the reality of your life, your mind deals with ideas about life.*

The next chapter explores how to meditate without an object—it's meditating on space.

Chapter 15: Meditating on space

Space doesn't have a shape or colour; you can't hear it, smell it or touch it. And yet nothing could exist without it. Everything we experience is dependent on space.

Space is something we never think about. When I'm teaching, I like to ask people what they noticed when they came into the room. Naturally they point out what they have seen—chairs, carpets, tables, pictures, lights, the other people, colours, books, CDs and so on.

No-one ever mentions space, which isn't surprising because we can't actually see it. It doesn't have a shape or colour; you can't hear it, smell it or touch it. And yet without space there wouldn't be any room for things to have their own shape. Space is the ingredient that gives everything a place and keeps it in that place; it's the matrix in which everything exists.

Space is a key object for meditation. It shifts the focus of your meditation away from the objects you would normally use to the space around them. This changes your perspective so that, instead of looking at things, you are looking at their context—the edges of things and what lies between them. For example, you can see the beginning and end of each thought and each breath, and learn to hold your focus on the space between you and what you would normally look at.

Meditating on space can therefore be used to develop the quality of "just watching", which allows you to become aware that everything comes and goes. This chapter explores meditating on space; you will find practical instructions for meditating formally and informally on space at the end of the chapter.

Space is always there

If you look at the room you are in, you will notice that space in the room is the only thing that stays constant. Everything else can be moved around, eventually falls apart and is thrown away. This is another reason we don't notice space—it doesn't really change. We only notice things that move.

When you meditate on space you are meditating on *no object*—you can't see it because it doesn't move. Like a room where we notice the things and not the space they exist in, we only notice the thoughts, images and conversations in our minds. It doesn't occur to us that there is anything else, because we can't see or hear it. Thoughts, images and conversations come and go, they have shape, colour and sound—so we notice them. However, without space they could not exist. So in your mind, as in the world around you, space is the essential ingredient that allows everything else to exist.

We get trapped in our thoughts and inner conversations because they are always moving. They drag us along with them and we can't get out. It's exhausting when you feel this is all there is—a continuous stream that carries you along whether you like it or not.

So we try to pin thoughts down. Hold onto images. Keep repeating conversation. And eventually find that this is even more exhausting because it is utterly impossible. We have an instinct there must be something else—something permanent, unchanging—but we have no idea where to look, so spend an enormous amount of time and energy trying to keep ideas, images and the things around us permanent. Only to find it doesn't work.

The space in our minds

The space in our mind is the foundation of our mind. It is a state of awareness—a clear, open, vivid state of mind that is there all the time, whether you are thinking or not. It's what you discover when you are "just watching" something, and find you can stay in that state whether the object you are watching stays there or not.

A child can rest in awareness easily when they become totally absorbed in something, stay completely still and just watch. Children often "space out" but unfortunately we gradually train ourselves to stop this, so end up ignoring space completely.

As you re-train yourself to *just watch*, you become increasingly aware of the space around what you are watching. You don't become so caught by things you normally focus on, because you see that they all come and go. In the same way that everything exists in a matrix of space, everything in your mind exists in a matrix of awareness. This fundamental quality of awareness is always there.

Informal meditations on space

Initially, meditations on space are designed to lead you to become aware of the space around you. You can then open your mind to it, notice the space when you are outside and get the feel of it. Here are a range of informal meditations on space.

Feel and notice the space around you

Feeling the breeze on your skin is a good way to begin to notice space.

> Begin by noticing the feel of the air moving over your skin, so that you are focusing on the air itself. As you focus on the air around you, open your mind to the space around you, so you become aware, for example, of the space in parks, by the sea, in streets and buildings.

Meditate on the sky

Meditating on the sky is an excellent way to meditate on space.

A psychologist friend said this meditation changed her life because it allowed her to let go of everything she had to deal with during the day. By focusing on the sky she could free her mind and open up the space in her mind.

The night sky

Meditating on the night sky is an incredibly beautiful way to meditate on space.

> Take a rug outside and lay on your back on the ground so you can open your mind to the vast, open sky, filled with stars. It's an incredible feeling and provides a sense of how our own planet exists in space.

Formal meditations on space

Formal meditations on space are designed to open you to the space in your mind, and lead you to understand that this space is actually a state of awareness that is always there.

There are a number of formal meditations for meditating on space.

Noticing the ends of thoughts

If while meditating, you notice that your thoughts have slowed down, you can turn to meditating on space by becoming aware of the end of each thought.

> Rocking, Bodycheck, Sound
>
> When a thought ends, instead of looking for the next one, or returning to your meditation object, just rest there and notice what it feels like.
>
> Explore the quality that is left in your mind when the thought stops.

Notice what it feels like when the next thought comes along.
Then become aware of the spaces between your thoughts.

Focusing on the end of the out-breath

You can also become aware of the end of each breath while meditating.

When you breathe out, let your mind rest there and notice what it feels like before you breathe in again.
Start to focus on this point at the end of each out-breath.

Noticing when sensations end

If you are meditating on the sensations in your body, you can do the same thing.

Notice the point at which each sensation ends and let your mind rest there, exploring the feeling of space.

Using a visual object

Meditating with your eyes open is a good way to meditate on space.

Rocking, Bodycheck, Sound
Begin meditating with a visual object (see instructions in Chapter 4). When you have established calm and concentration, let the focus of your eyes come back to rest half-way between you and the object. You can then let your mind rest on the space between yourself and the object.

Meditating directly on space

You can also meditate directly on space.

Rocking, Bodycheck, Sound
Look at the wall in front of you.
Half-close your eyes and soften your focus, and allow your focus to shift to the point half-way between yourself and the wall. You will notice everything in your line of vision but it will go into the background, and the space in front of you will become your meditation object.
(You can practice this informally just by looking at things, then shifting your focus to the space between yourself and the object and letting your mind rest there for a while.)

Every time I return to the Lifeflow retreat centre I notice my mind opening up, because I am moving from the tight, ordered spaces of the city, to the wide open space of the country. As you practise this, you can begin to feel your awareness expand.

Meditating on space, then, is a key meditation for learning how to become aware of the space in your own mind. These meditations are particularly effective while on retreat, and retreat work is the focus of the next chapter.

Chapter 16: **Advanced retreat**

Your retreat work nourishes your daily life, and your daily practice sustains your retreat work.

Getting the balance right in retreat is essential. Many people have bad retreat experiences through pushing so hard that their body breaks down, or the retreat becomes so rarefied they completely lose contact with reality. It's important to remember that nearly all the classical rules for retreat come from a monastic tradition where the monks led a specialised life with nothing else to do.

Retreat experience can be so divorced from everyday life that it remains separate from it and becomes idealised. Instead of being a fulfilling learning experience that nourishes your life, it can leave you feeling intensely frustrated. When you are doing more advanced retreats it's therefore useful to structure them so that what you do in retreat can be integrated with your everyday life.

There are many retreat practices which can be carried over to your daily meditation practice. For example, mantras and visualisations can be developed to a high degree in retreat, but can also be done in everyday life more informally. Just repeating them keeps your mind in a calm, balanced state while walking, driving and doing routine tasks. You are then at least aware of the conversation in your head! It is an easy way to sustain the calm of retreat in your daily life.

Then the daily meditation practice you maintain—whether it be ten minutes or one hour per day—sustains your retreat experience. When you are able to do more retreat work, you will find that you can pick up at the point you left off in your last retreat.

This chapter explores the different types of retreats and outlines how experienced meditators can use retreats as an integral part of their practice.

The different types of retreats

Although you can keep the same basic routine during retreat, it can be adapted, and will vary considerably depending on which type of retreat you are doing. Each type of retreat—Calm and Concentration, Insight, Tantra and informal—has its own aims and develops its own flavour.

Calm and Concentration

In a retreat dedicated to developing Calm and Concentration, you develop the ability to hold your body relaxed and your mind and emotions calm and balanced through all four meditation postures—sitting, standing, walking and lying down—and during every activity. You can hold a reasonably balanced state from the moment you wake up to the moment you go to sleep.

A Calm and Concentration retreat also enables you to:

1. restore your energies and develop your sense of emotional and mental balance. This gives you the resources and ability to maintain your physical, emotional and mental health throughout all the different conditions of your daily life.

2. explore and become skillful in reaching the deepening levels of meditation. You learn how to recognise and hold them and this gives you the ability to develop real mental strength and stability.

3. explore the different categories of meditation—the kinds of meditations you wouldn't normally experience in depth.

Exploring different meditations in a Calm and Concentration retreat broadens your repertoire. You know which kinds of meditations suit you, but exploring a wider range, although you may not be so proficient at them, can open aspects of yourself you would otherwise have ignored.

For example, I have never been particularly good at visualisations, but when I started to focus on them they opened up a vivid palette of colours in my mind which I had never noticed before. I had hardly been aware of colour, both in my mind and in the world around me.

Another example is meditating on death, which few people choose to focus on. Yet whenever we hold retreats which involve meditating on something that has died, the effect is totally unexpected. Everyone finds that there is no fear, just a deep feeling of peace and stillness. They also find, to their surprise, that it opens their hearts to a sense of warmth and understanding they could never have predicted.

Insight

One major purpose of retreat is to reduce external input to your senses so you can focus on and learn about your own thoughts, emotions and body. Insight retreat specialises in reducing this input to an absolute minimum. I liken it to scientific laboratory work where you work in a closely controlled environment to examine reactions to particular situations.

In Insight meditation you concentrate on seeing and experiencing how your mind, thoughts and emotions work, how they affect the way you perceive the world, and what human consciousness is like. You aim to bring your mind to the point where it is completely balanced and still, using meditations for calm and concentration. Insight adds the dimension of becoming aware of this state *while you are in it*, to see and experience what the mind is like when it is still. Your focus moves away from meditating on something outside, to your mind itself. It's like being at the cinema, then stopping watching the film, and turning around so that you see the light and the projector. This is not easy, because we normally either "clock off" at this point, or go to sleep.

There are five distinct levels of insight into the mind. Four of these are developed in Insight meditation and the fifth is realised as part of the meditative stream of Tantra. They enable you to see and experience your mind when it is still, how thoughts work and what they are; the relationship between your mind, body and the world; and how concepts shape your perceptions. (These levels of insight are explored in detail in my book *Insight and Love*.)

The fifth level of insight, an integral part of Tantra, is the experience of the fact that your mind, or consciousness itself, is luminous. This means it is vibrant and alive even when resting in its foundation state of pure awareness, when it is not moving with thoughts or emotions. You discover that the "space" in your mind is not dull or dark but living and radiant with energy.

Tantra

A retreat concentrating on Tantra is very different from an Insight or Calm and Concentration retreat. Working with Tantra is very dynamic; it's a thorough emotional workout.

The yoga-tantras are a series of exercises designed to open up your inner world. They are given the name *yoga* because they work in exactly the same way as physical yoga. They stretch and loosen your inner body; called your *energy body* in the tantric tradition, which consists of the sensations, emotions, visions and sounds that make up our inner life.

You begin by creating an internal structure. Like all structures it is fairly arbitrary but absolutely necessary. For example, in sport, the size of the playing field needs to be defined otherwise it is impossible to play the game—the line needs to be drawn. In Tantra this line is drawn through the centre of the body, from the top of the head to the pit of the abdomen. It's a way to define the balance point of all our inner experiences— where everything is at rest.

Imagine any emotion or inner sensation swinging from side to side, left to right. It could be smooth and gentle or wild and erratic. Like a pendulum, it will eventually slow down and come to rest, and this resting point will be at the line through the centre of the body. This is where we will feel calm, relaxed and "centred".

However, there is another plane to be taken into account. This is the polarity we experience between the head and the groin—from the top of the line to the bottom. Sensations can swing up and down as well as from side to side, so the balance point for this plane is the heart centre, at the centre of the line.

Energy
Rising

Energy
Sinking

Having established an internal structure, Tantra provides a way to consciously create vibrant and healthy emotional states by integrating the wild emotions we are generally afraid of: for example, the extreme ecstasy of feeling alive through every cell of our bodies, the youthful bliss of sexuality, passionate involvement with something we care deeply about, outrage at injustice. (Often we either repress or indulge these wild emotions when unconscious—drunk or drugged in some way.)

Tantra also explores the states we pass through as we fall asleep and experience in deep sleep; the aim is to be aware right through

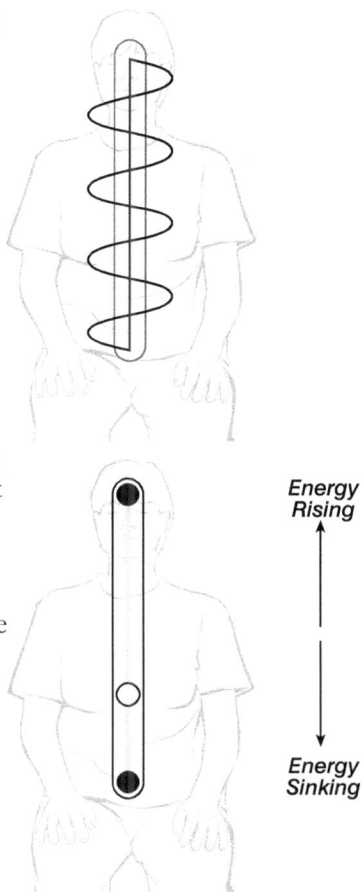

these stages. There is also an exercise for remaining conscious while dreaming, and one for exploring our perceptions—of ourselves, our bodies and everything else. Tantra also opens up the process of dying, because it is possible to consciously pass through all the stages the mind goes through when it approaches death.

Some of these tantric exercises are immediately applicable to our daily lives, and once learned can become an extremely valuable tool. However, many can only be practised under retreat conditions because they require a degree of calm and concentration that can't be attained while our energies are being used up in everyday life.

These exercises are invaluable for experiencing and therefore understanding some of the big questions about our lives—who we are, what our emotions are, and what death is actually like. They take the fear out of many things that drive and worry us at a subliminal level. Carl Jung acknowledged the wisdom of the Tibetan tantric approach to death in his commentary to *The Tibetan Book of the Dead*[12].

Informal retreats

Informal retreats are an ideal way to train yourself to maintain awareness no matter what you are doing. My teacher focused on this a lot. For example, at a retreat in Assisi where I had been meditating in a very concentrated way for some time, he arrived at the house without any warning and asked me to drive someone immediately to Sienna.

I was shocked as I believed that if I broke my retreat routine I would lose the calm and concentration completely. However, I did what was asked, and learned one of the most important lessons of my life concerning meditation and retreat. I found that, in spite of my concerns about suddenly being pitched into driving in heavy traffic, I had no problems whatsoever. I was able to remain completely calm and focused—dealing with traffic and having to move quickly made no difference to my state of mind. Most surprising was that when I returned I could pick up my retreat work exactly where I left off without any detrimental effect—in fact, I felt fresher and clearer. My teacher smiled.

People are often afraid of "losing it" if they do not keep strictly to their retreat routine. However, this ensures that what is experienced in retreat never becomes part of daily life. Informal retreats are an excellent way to integrate the focused calm of retreat with the busyness of everyday life.

An informal retreat is more appropriate if you have a reasonably long time available, for example, one to six months. It is set up so that you concentrate on retreat work for most of the time, but include things you need to do to keep your daily life intact. For example, some of my students have spent a day or two each week in town keeping up with work or study. Others have brought their work to the retreat centre so that they can spend an hour or so each day focusing on it.

I liken this process to learning to change gears in a car: to moving at different speeds efficiently. We tend to experience only two gears––we are either busy or asleep—and we never learn how to move smoothly from one to the other. In informal retreat, you learn to move effortlessly from being still and focused, to dealing with what has to be done, without losing your awareness. You can keep your mind calm and focused and your body reasonably relaxed while meditating, walking, driving, having a conversation, playing sport, studying, dealing with work issues and so on.

You learn to become aware of every emotion and thought that arises, instead of trying to hold on to some and ignoring the rest. You no longer need to be afraid of emotions and situations you don't like or don't feel capable of dealing with, because you have space to become used to them and accept them, and see what part they play in your life. So you can keep yourself calm and clear no matter what is happening.

Lifeflow members' retreats

Retreats for Lifeflow members focus on particular aspects of one of the four streams of the meditation tradition (Calm and Concentration, Insight, Tantra and Ethics), so that members can develop a good experiential understanding of the material contained in them. They run from four to ten days.

They are directed lightly with three guided sessions a day. In the morning there is a class focusing on the theme of the retreat, in the afternoon a deep relaxation session, and a guided meditation in the evening. They are structured so that members have plenty of time to practise on their own.

Those members who wish to train to become a senior teacher are required to do a year-long retreat. This provides space and time to focus on Insight meditation and Tantra, and so fully integrate these practices into daily life. A retreat of a year's duration provides the opportunity for someone to become aware of, and experience, the whole cycle of nature at it passes through four seasons—a chance to feel the connection of your body with the earth.

The aim of this is to change the foundation of your life from ideas and beliefs, to one that is resting in the reality of the body and its life on this planet. This is a profound shift. It means you can live grounded in the reality of your body and its relationship with nature. Instead of being directed by the ideas and forces that drive us all, you can be truly inner-directed—keeping in touch with your inner sensations and the core of your being.

A year in retreat

My first year in retreat proved to be a complete turning point because I found that, after spending three years living in Paris, my body was running on adrenalin. It took a month or so to get through the withdrawal and discover what it was like to live each day completely in touch with my body.

The retreat was held in Assisi, Italy, an incredibly beautiful place, in an old farmhouse in the country surrounded by the rich landscape of small farms, vines and large stands of trees. Around the house lived geese, ducks, turkeys, hens, a cow and an enormous pig. Every day we had fresh eggs from the hens and milk from the cow. The house itself was the centre of all activities in the neighbourhood and each year everyone gathered there, with great ceremony, to press the year's harvest of grapes and make wine.

One day while meditating I felt myself literally sinking into the earth. It was as though I was being embraced by it, held and drawn into it. My body opened and softened as it sank deeper and deeper—I felt as though I was floating in the earth. It was an indescribably blissful experience.

The embrace I experienced was warm and nourishing and I could feel my body being sustained by it. The Italian earth was rich and dark, and in meditation it felt like dark chocolate. This was my first experience of being in union with the earth and it totally changed my relationship with the natural world. I realised how intimately our bodies are united with nature. St Francis of Assisi was part of the nature mysticism tradition, and sang of Brother Sun and Sister Moon[13]. He saw, as anyone who opens to this experience must see, that all the animals, birds and plants on this earth, and all the stars and planets that surround us, are part of one enormous family.

As I sank into the earth I felt that it was, in a very real sense, the mother of our bodies. My body was held and nourished by the earth as though I was being held in its arms. I could feel right through my body exactly what St Francis meant; why he could so happily talk to birds and animals—and why they understood him. Indigenous people of Australia completely understand this, because they feel this country to be their mother. When I returned to Australia I discovered a new country.

Our bodies are born from the earth so our lives are intimately embedded in the rhythms and cycles of nature. Unfortunately, our lifestyle prohibits most of us from experiencing this. However, in retreat you have the time and space to open your senses and feel the life around you in all its miraculous variety. You can actually feel the spirit of the natural world through your entire body as your senses open to the sights, sounds, smells, tastes and touch of nature. As the breeze caresses your skin, the light and colours fill your mind, and the smells of trees and flowers and sounds of birds soak through your body, you feel the ecstasy of coming home.

Over the year in retreat I could also feel the changes from season to season and how our bodies respond to these. I discovered the profound calm and awareness of the subconscious mind and how being open to it keeps you peaceful, vibrant and alert. When you are in touch with your body you live far more efficiently because you are not fighting yourself to maintain a way of life that is ultimately unsustainable.

Retreat also provides the perfect environment for exploring your emotions in much greater depth. The next chapter explores how you can use retreat time to penetrate and transform emotions.

Chapter 17: Observing and letting go of emotions in retreat

As you observe your body in retreat you find that emotions are completely misunderstood.

In retreat you can study in more detail what emotions are and how they work; it's a further extension of the **Three C Technique**.

The reason for observing emotions is to free yourself from believing the stories that have been built up around them. You discover that emotions are not what you think they are, and you can see unhealthy emotions coming long before they hit you, so you have the ability to step aside and let them pass.

Developing this skill is important because you need to feel confident that you won't get caught in the particular emotion you are working with. I recommend the guidance of a teacher for this. Use the first day or two in retreat just to establish calm and concentration. Once you have settled in, a habitual emotion may surface which you can work with, and emotions will arise simply through interacting and living with other people.

This chapter outlines the procedure for working with an emotion in retreat: from accepting and coming to know it, to experiencing it in your body so you can penetrate to the core of it. You will find the practical instructions for letting go of emotions in retreat at the end of the chapter.

Accepting what you are feeling

Because many people are afraid to allow themselves to feel strongly, the first step is to **Catch the moment** and accept whatever it is you are feeling—anger, fear, wanting, anxiety, aggression, lust, yearning, loneliness or grief, to name just a few. You might even be experiencing joy or ecstasy.

> My composition teacher in Paris was fiercely attacked early in his life because his music was so unashamedly ecstatic. The audience at the time, and particularly the critics, were outraged because it wasn't polite or cerebral. It was so energetic, colourful and exciting that the first time I heard it I burst out laughing, lay on the floor and kicked my legs in the air. They accused him of being a psychopath and he was forbidden to teach composition

at the Paris Conservatoire for years. Obviously they assumed that decent, respectable people didn't have such feelings—because *they* certainly didn't—or didn't allow themselves to experience them. It's sad how common this is.

Allow yourself to feel the emotion. The temptation to censor or diminish it in some way, to try and solve it or make a production of it, may be very strong, so keep your mind with your body, just staying with the feeling. "Expressing" emotions—acting them out in the theatre of your ego—can be just another way of running away from actually feeling them in your body.

Because emotions are such powerful forces, there may be fear attached to what you are feeling and if so, stay with that too. You may feel indulgent, but you are giving your *body* time to talk to you, instead of controlling and constricting its world and its language. Retreat provides the ideal conditions for this. When the body, or subconscious mind, is speaking, it is unsophisticated, it takes time, and it is direct. So it takes a while to learn the language.

You might have found it helpful to name what you are feeling when using this technique at home (as outlined in Chapter 8) but in retreat I would suggest not naming it—just allow yourself to *rest* with the feeling. When you name something you place it in the library of your past experience—your memories—and relate it to what you already know. So if you can explore something in retreat, it is much more effective if you *don't* name what is happening.

Let yourself "not know" what is happening

This brings us to the second stage of **Clear the space**. By staying with your meditation exercise, you can maintain your balance in the face of strong emotions, and just watch what is happening in your body. Let yourself rest in the open space of "not knowing"—what a mediaeval mystic called *The Cloud of Unknowing*[14].

When we are learning something new or opening to a new experience, we often want to know what is going to happen before it happens. However, if we did know, it wouldn't be a new experience! It would be a memory of something we had already experienced. Let your body take you where it needs to go, rather than you directing what it is doing.

For many people this is overwhelming because it's a process of learning to trust what you have been taught *not* to trust. You have caught the wave of the emotion, you are on it, and now you are learning to ride it by staying completely still.

You are safe because you are in retreat, no-one else is involved, and each time you feel you've had enough, you can just stop the meditation session and the experience will stop too. It's as though your body knows that you will return when the space is there to allow things to surface.

Experiencing your body on its own terms

You are now ready to **Change the habit**. Having the opportunity in retreat to rest with an emotion rather than trying to work out, or assuming you know what it is, allows you to experience it on its own terms. You are in touch with the actual sensations in your body instead of interpreting them through thinking.

Every time your mind goes back to thinking about the emotion, or what has caused it, or trying to solve it and get rid of it, gently bring it back to the actual sensations in your body. Focus directly on the sensations and explore them. Discover what you *are* feeling, instead of what you think you are feeling. Encourage the feelings and let them grow; allow the sensations to fill your focus and your mind.

Your body might start to move around, stretch, arch or double up, or it might remain perfectly still. You might start to cry, moan or laugh. Just let it all happen and allow your body to have its say. All you have to do is observe, and not get caught in what you think might, should, or could be happening. Just stay with what *is* happening.

Eventually, any reactions to what you are feeling will settle, and you will return to stillness. Don't try to force this; your body will follow its own cycle, and by staying with it you can learn what this cycle is and see how it unfolds.

The core of emotions

Now you can see what is at the core of the emotion you are experiencing; the sensations in your body are like currents in the sea or movements of wind on the earth. They are simply there, and are your body's natural and immediate response to what is happening. Our bodies respond to every sense stimulus, external or internal, whether from our senses or from the ideas, thoughts and images in our minds. The *experience* of sensations is very clear and direct.

How you *interpret* this is another thing entirely and depends on your memories and past experience. Usually we have never experienced this distinction, so it's no wonder we are in the dark about our emotional and instinctual world.

It's not the physical experience that creates a problem—it's when you name an emotion and start to think about it that conflict arises. Your conscious mind goes round and round the same emotion, even though it might be long gone, trying to fit it into the bank of memories that make up your identity. It reviews your past experience, what you were taught you should feel, what you expect to feel, and your plans for the future, to see if it can be slotted into any of these. So you are focused on an *interpretation* of past events and ideas, whether you are aware of this or not. The conflict and pain arise because this interpretation is not in line with what is actually happening now; you are not focused on the direct experience of your body. *Your body cannot remain in the past—it is only ever in the present.*

As you sit with the direct experience of your body you will become very calm, and will discover the energy at the core of the emotion, and that is all it is—*energy*. It can take different forms as it moves through the body in particular ways, just like currents and winds. For example, desire is the life energy of the body—powerful, surging, urging it to live and grow. At the core of anger is crystal clarity; the drive to distinguish things clearly and accurately so we can see exactly what is happening.

At the centre of every emotion is a deep stillness from which the movement of the emotion arises. Learning to be still with emotions takes the fear out of them. They are our means of survival—the powerful forces that direct our bodies. Fear will change to awe and understanding as you are increasingly able to feel the direct movements of energy in your body.

Hanging on to the names for emotions creates chaos until you open to the experience of your body. You can then create a new name from your own bodily experience rather than what you were taught in the past. You can reshape your habits and actions because you are aware of what you are doing and *how you are feeling in your body* as you do it.

The first time I experienced this, I had decided to just sit with the desire I was feeling instead of using meditation to calm it down. It became overwhelming, a feeling of intense yearning which literally took over my whole body, knotting it up completely. There wasn't even an object to yearn for—just this incredibly painful emotion.

Then it turned into anger, and eventually a profound sense of loneliness. Finally, my mind and body became completely still and I could feel a warm, flickering, luminous feeling right through my body. I realised I had "come home". If I had believed the stories associated with any of these emotions, I would have been stuck. All the pain and desire came from believing my ideas about what *should* be happening instead of being completely in touch with my body.

When you let go of your ideas you discover the life in your own body—you are directly in touch with it, instead of searching for a feeling of being alive everywhere else.

Instructions for observing emotions in retreat

Catch the moment

Accept what you are feeling.

Allow yourself to stay with the feeling without censoring or naming it. If you are fearful, stay with that too. Don't try to do anything about what is happening.

Clear the space

Rest in the open space of "not-knowing". Simply keep focused on your meditation and the sensations in your body, using them as an anchor.

Let your body take you where it needs to go, rather than you directing what it does. Stay still and ride the wave.

When you feel you've had enough, just stop the meditation session and take a break.

Change the habit

Every time your mind returns to thinking about the emotion, gently bring it back to focus on the actual sensations in your body—notice where they are and explore them.

Allow the sensations to fill your focus and mind.

Your body might start to move around, stretch, arch or double up or stay still. You might start to cry, moan or laugh. Just let it all happen; allow your body to have its say.

Just watch, and observe everything that is happening.

See what is at the core of the emotion you are experiencing.

As you do this, images, memories, conversations and thoughts associated with the emotion may arise. It's useful to write them down after the meditation session or draw an image of the emotion in colour, as vividly as you can. These images and thoughts can be very accurate, and once they are allowed into your awareness, the knot associated with them has the chance to let go.

If you had been ill or in an accident, one of the essential conditions for recovery is that you allow yourself to feel tired so the body can concentrate on healing itself. Emotions follow the same patterns as the physical body. One of the major signs of transforming an emotion and letting a knot go is a sense of tiredness. It's that very deep, satisfying tiredness that comes from the relief of being able to give up something that has been a burden for some time. The mind and body have a chance to adjust and regroup their resources, because the energy that has been locked up is available for redistribution in a healthier, happier and more balanced way.

Retreat is also an ideal time to fine-tune your meditation by becoming aware of whether your mind is too tight or too loose, and practise using techniques to adjust the balance. The next chapter explores this topic in detail.

Chapter 18: Fine-tuning your meditation

As your meditation practice develops you can fine-tune your focus by being aware without thinking.

Chapter 3 briefly outlined how you can tune your meditation by becoming aware of whether your mind is too tight or too loose. This chapter discusses in detail how you can *fine*-tune your meditation––recognise when your mind and emotions are in or out of balance and maintain your balance while meditating. The instructions in this chapter are aimed at retreat practice, when your body is refreshed, rather than everyday meditating. They become particularly relevant as your practice progresses and you develop the ability to hold the different levels of absorption.

Usually when you are too focused on thinking your mind becomes too tight as your body becomes tense; here you are ignoring the subconscious mind, and therefore the feelings and emotions in your body. When you are too focused on your feelings your mind becomes too loose; here you are ignoring the conscious mind, as you drift into the wash of feelings that pass through your body without discriminating between them.

Because the foundation of both the subconscious and conscious minds is awareness, our subconscious mind (instincts and emotions) is as aware as our thinking. For our bodies to respond to immediate sensory input, they have to be aware of the sensation. In the same way, to communicate emotionally, there has to be awareness. We have become so used to equating *consciousness* with thinking and self-consciousness, we have forgotten that our minds and bodies also have to be aware of instincts and emotions to survive. So, in a very real sense, our bodies are conscious, whether we, as part of the conversation in our heads that sees us in *here* and everything else as out *there*, are aware of it or not.

This kind of awareness does not register as thinking, but as feeling, and meditation enables you to access and understand it. This is important because when it comes to tuning the balance of your mind, you can't do it through thinking, it's something you come to know through feeling. You become aware of whether your mind is too tight or too loose by feeling the effect of this *in your emotions and in your body.*

People tune an engine or a guitar by listening—using the direct awareness of their senses, not by thinking about it. In the same way, you tune the balance of your mind by listening to your body and opening to the sensations in your head, heart and gut.

Recognising when your mind is too tight

If you become too tight you will be agitated and anxious and begin to get frustrated with your meditation. You will become physically tense and will probably be trying too hard; your mind will jump around so much that it cannot settle in one place. Habitual worries and concerns will take over and your mind will get caught in its cage of thought.

Posture

In this agitated state you have completely lost touch with the feelings and sensations of your body, so to balance your mind, you need to relax your posture so you can begin to feel again.

> Allow your jaw to drop slightly so that your top and bottom teeth are apart but you can still keep your lips together.
> Check that your shoulders are relaxed. Let them drop slightly as you relax the shoulder muscles.
> Feel your chest and open it, then move to the abdomen and loosen the muscles there.

If you find that you need to do something more active, do the Spot Meditation Contact Points but deliberately tense each of these parts of your body, and then relax them by letting go as follows.

> Feel the contact of your feet on the floor, your thighs on the chair, your backside on the chair, your back on the backrest, and your arms and hands on your thighs, lap or arm rests of the chair.
> Now, move your awareness back to your left foot, tighten it, then let go and allow it to sink into the floor.
> Now tense your right foot, then let go and allow it sink into the floor.
> Tense your left thigh, then let go and allow it to sink into the chair, then do the same with your right thigh.
> Tense the muscles of your backside, then let go and allow it to sink into the chair.

Feel your back on the backrest and tense the muscles then let go, and let yourself have the feeling of slightly falling back into the chair. Finally, tense the muscles of your arms and hands then let go and allow them to rest into your thighs or lap, feeling the weight of your hands resting on your legs or arms of the chair.

There are many other ways to relax your muscles; one of the most effective ways is to use the beginning of the Mind and Body Washing Meditation (outlined in full in Chapter 4).

Imagine yourself outside in a warm, sunny place so that you can feel the warmth of the air on your skin.

Gently allow this warmth to soak into all the muscles of your body, starting at the top of the head, moving down to the face and over the whole head, the neck, throat, shoulders, arms and hands.

Then allow the warmth to gently soak into the muscles of your chest and upper back, your stomach and the middle of the back, your abdomen, hips, lower back and backside.

And finally allow the warmth to soak into the muscles of your legs and feet.

Eyes

If you try too hard to meditate you often stare, even with your eyes closed—looking straight ahead and forcing yourself to concentrate. We all learned to concentrate in this way and it is very counterproductive.

When you are too tense you will probably be doing this. To overcome it:

If you are meditating with your eyes closed, open them, and look about a metre in front of you.

Then lower your focus, keeping it below the horizontal and gently close your eyes again or, if you prefer, leave them half-open.

Simply becoming aware of where your eyes are focused, and gently lowering your focus with your eyes still closed may be enough. If your eyes are literally darting around all over the place, do the following:

Gently massage the muscles around your eyes to help ease the tension.

Visualise a deep blue light at the pit of your stomach—it moves the focus of your gaze deeper into your body.

Tongue

When you are too tight, your tongue is usually pressed hard against your top teeth.

Gently and deliberately place the tip of your tongue behind the bottom teeth to help re-establish a calm and balanced state.

Breathing

Your breathing will become shallow, fast and sharp when you are too tight. To balance this:

Follow your in-breath right down to the abdomen and when you breathe out, imagine the breath spreading through your whole body.

Feel it soaking into all the muscles and organs, and then imagine it leaving through the skin. Do this for a few breaths until you feel more balanced.

Also become aware of the movement of your abdomen as you breathe and rest your awareness there, watching and feeling it rising and falling to help you re-establish calm.

Generally

When you become "tight" while meditating, you may feel too agitated to continue. In this case, the best thing to do is stop the meditation session. One of the key factors in tense agitation is either neglecting the body or pushing it too hard.

Use the rest of the time you had set aside for meditation to do some physical exercise—something that gets your breathing going so you work and tire your muscles.

Recognising when your mind is too loose

If your mind is too loose, you tend to become dull or dazed. Your mind drifts off and starts to wander aimlessly without you being aware of where it has gone. It tends to go down very well-worn tracks, drifting into the habitual fantasies that live in the dark, backstage recesses of your mind. It feels as though you are sinking into a deep trough.

You might also go into a haze, where your senses are blurred and you feel drugged. This is the dreamy, glazed-eyed, "spacey" state that every send-up of meditation impersonates.

You may also drift off to sleep. If so, there is no need for concern because it means your body is tired and needs rest. It is easy to distinguish between going to sleep or into a state of absorption. If your head does not drop forward (so your chin is on your chest), you did not go to sleep no matter what it felt like.

Posture

When your mind is too loose your body starts to slump, so a good way to tighten concentration is to check your posture.

> Run your awareness through your body, checking your head, shoulders, arms and hands, stomach, legs, knees and feet.
>
> Check that your spine is erect, and that the back of your neck feels open with your chin very slightly tucked in.
>
> If you are sitting in a chair, check that your knees are almost at right angles. Ensure that your knees are apart and the soles of your feet are firmly on the floor so that your hips are stable.
>
> Become aware of the position of your hands; hold them in the lap with the left hand under the right, or rest them, palms down, on your thighs.

Eyes

You can also fine-tune your mind by noticing where your eyes are focused. As you relax they will lower, even if they are closed, and as your concentration sharpens they lift. So if your mind becomes too loose, lifting the focus of your eyes can help sharpen it.

> Slightly lift the focus of your eyes, keeping them just below the horizontal.
>
> Visualise a white light at the centre of your forehead to help lift the focus of your gaze and lighten the feeling-tone of your mind.

If you lift your eyes above the horizontal, your mind will become too sharp—this posture is used for Insight meditation practice because it deliberately sharpens your mind to "wake up" the calm.

As you develop your meditation practice, you may find that keeping your eyes closed can contribute to drowsiness.

If your mind becomes too loose, open your eyes, look up, then lower your gaze so you are slightly looking down and close them again.

You might prefer to leave your eyes open. If so:

Allow your eyes to soften by letting the eyelids drop half-way.

Let your gaze rest about a metre in front of you, then let your focus drop so that it's just below horizontal.

Tongue

Another fine-tuning technique is to check the position of your tongue. If your mind is becoming too loose:

Lift the tip of your tongue to rest for a while behind your top teeth to sharpen your focus.

When you feel more balanced, place it back behind the bottom teeth.

Breathing

As you become drowsier your breathing will become slower and heavier. If you notice this:

Move your awareness to your nostrils, watching and feeling the breath entering and leaving your body.

You can also sharpen your mind by imagining breathing into your head.

Breathe in and follow the breath through to the centre of your chest.

When you breathe out, focus the out-breath into your head. You may feel your head becoming lighter and more spacious. Do this for a few breaths, and check if this has freshened your state of mind.

Another breathing technique for when you become too loose is to place your awareness at your nostrils. Then:

Feel each in-breath move up to the top of the nose, and when you can feel this, follow the breath into your head.

You may be able to feel the breath expanding through your head, freshening and clearing it.

Generally

Check that your room isn't too warm and stuffy; it should be fresh and airy. If all else fails, break your meditation session. Washing your face with cold water might refresh you enough to continue, or it might be better to walk outside then try meditating later.

Maintaining balance while meditating

One of the best ways to sustain a calm, alert state of mind—not too tight or too loose—is to keep your meditation sessions short and frequent. Many people think that if they meditate for a longer time they achieve more from it but this isn't necessarily so.

When you meditate beyond where your mind is capable of holding concentration you enter a slightly dozy, drifting, unaware state. If your meditation is boring your mind will wander off to something else anyway. At best it's a bit relaxing; at worst it's a waste of time. To maintain the quality of your meditation it is far better to work within the limits of your mind and body so you come to know their rhythms and cycles.

Keeping your meditation sessions short and frequent keeps them fresh, keeps your interest there and ensures they don't become boring. It's also much easier to achieve, which makes it easier to build in the habit of practising.

Bliss, clarity and connection

When your mind and emotions are balanced, thoughts and feelings still come and go, but they flow smoothly through your awareness without getting stuck. They pass by like a gentle breeze, and you can just watch them without getting involved in any way.

Every so often you will enter the deeper levels of absorption—the second, third and fourth levels—where initially your thoughts, and then the feelings and sensations you experience, will come to rest and pause for a while. When this happens, your body, emotions and mind have become completely balanced, and you experience **bliss, clarity** and **connection**. These are definite signs of having established a calm and concentrated state of mind. In the meditation tradition they are called *the three gifts*, because they feel so wonderful.

Bliss—a balanced body

The first quality is **bliss**. An athlete wouldn't work so hard if somewhere along the line it didn't feel good, and working from this physically balanced state is like dancing, or driving a well-oiled, smooth-running car. It's blissful. You feel truly in your body—no longer caught in thoughts—and you can feel the sensations and energies flowing smoothly and freely.

Bliss can be anything from a quiet, self-contained sense of joy to ecstatic rapture where you feel so full of energy and feeling that you wonder if you can contain it without exploding.

Clarity—balanced emotions

The second quality is **clarity**. Instead of emotions churning, knotting, getting stuck, and crashing through your body, they settle into their natural, balanced state. There is no underlying state of emotional conflict because your emotions become still and calm, and when this happens you become very clear.

A traditional comparison to describe this is what happens with muddy water. As long as the water keeps moving and churning around, it stays muddy. But when the water becomes still the mud gradually settles and the water becomes clear, so you can see straight through it.

Clarity, then, is a sign that your emotions have settled so your mind becomes like a still, clear lake reflecting everything around it clearly.

Connection—a balanced mind

The third sign is **connection**. When thoughts are no longer passing through your mind, you see that its balanced state is spacious and completely open.

Because your mind is free of its incessant conversation and your body is free from the churning emotions that accompany this, you feel a sense of connection, as the separation you always feel when talking to yourself dissolves. You feel connected with your body, and have a sense of your *whole* body. You also feel connected with everything around you.

So these three signs—*bliss*, *clarity* and *connection*—are the qualities you experience when you have reached a completely balanced state. Your body feels blissful, your emotions have settled so you become clear, and your mind is open and connected with your body and the world around you.

Images of a balanced mind

There are a series of rather beautiful images from the meditation tradition, which describe a calm, concentrated and balanced state. (As images are the language of the body, you might find some of these arise spontaneously in your meditation when you reach this state.)

Sky and ocean

The sky and ocean have been used as images for the human mind. Like the mind, they can be calm and clear or stormy and cloudy. When they are free from clouds and waves, they both represent very accurately the mind when it is free from thoughts: balanced and still.

Space

Space is a strong image for a calm, clear mind, because it captures the sense of openness and infinity which arise when the conscious mind stops its chatter.

Light

Light is another common image to represent the mind. Tantric exercises are designed to reveal the *luminosity* of the mind, one of its main qualities. This experience arises when the mind is settled and completely balanced and you feel what it is like to experience the mind directly.

Crystal

The clarity of crystal is another classic image for the balanced mind. This also represents what the mind is like when free from thoughts. Like a diamond, its fundamental nature is completely clear, but can reflect all colours.

Classical images

The following images appear in the traditional texts—they are direct descriptions of a calm and concentrated state of mind, and also quite poetic[15].

- Like a cloudless sky, the sphere of your mind is broad and free.
- Like a waveless ocean, the mind is steady without thoughts.
- Like a bright lamp on a windless night, the consciousness is clear, bright and stable.
- A sphere that is vast like infinite space
- A mind steady as a mountain
- Pure consciousness, crystal clear and empty of thoughts

This chapter brings us to the close of Part Two. In Part Three we'll explore the philosophy and psychology of the meditation tradition, beginning with how to balance the conscious and subconscious parts of our minds.

Part Three: The theory behind the practice

Chapter 19: Balancing mind and body– the monkey and the elephant

The art of balance is knowing how and when to be still, and when to move.

While meditation is a tool for balancing yourself, physically, emotionally and mentally, anywhere, anytime, it doesn't mean always staying completely balanced, because then you would never be able to move. If you can find your balance point, you know where to start and finish any movement, whether physical or emotional.

This chapter explores the meaning of balance, the two minds and three levels of the brain, how these interact and how you can keep everything balanced.

Every athlete understands balance

Finding and maintaining physical balance is essential for athletes and sportspeople. Swimmers and runners in particular shake and move their bodies to warm and loosen up before a race, then stabilise and position themselves on the blocks. When you are measuring the outcome of a race in times of less than a second, how you line yourself up and that split second when you start, are crucial to the outcome.

If you are even slightly off-balance when you start, you will progressively lose your balance as you move. By the time you regain your balance, assuming that you do, you will have lost the race anyway. It's exactly the same emotionally.

Emotional and mental balance

If you are emotionally out of balance and do something in that state, you become further and further out of balance. The key to becoming aware of your emotional states and working with them skillfully is to know the point of emotional balance and be able to achieve it when you need to. The same applies mentally.

Much of our thinking is inefficient and unproductive, and this has profound implications, particularly in the workplace. Often when people are stressed or tired at work they push on, overriding the needs of their body. When you push hard, your work ceases to flow and, although you don't realise it, your thinking can become inefficient and the work often needs to be redone.

Our minds have a natural concentration span of 45–50 minutes, and when you learn to work within this, you can keep yourself fresh. Researchers have also found that our brains are programmed to have a short rest in the afternoon, which explains the drowsy feeling after lunch. It's a natural cycle of the brain.

Understanding these cycles and working with them instead of overriding them (as we are trained and expected to do), leads to more efficient use of our time and energies and a more enjoyable working life. We can recognise when our minds are balanced and linked with our bodies, and develop the skills to restore this balance quickly and easily. This ability can then be applied to every aspect of our lives.

An elite cricketer who began to see how much his state of mind affected his performance on the field told me, "I've trained my body and now I have to train my mind". After learning to use meditation he was delighted to achieve a hundred runs in an innings for the first time.

The two minds and three levels of the brain

According to Harvard psychologist Gregg Jacobs[16], the main cause for the overwhelming increase in stress, insomnia and depression in the last few decades is that we have completely overridden what he calls the *Ancestral Mind* with our *Thinking Mind*. Life is so bound up with the pressure of deadlines and information that pours in before we have time to process it and choose how to respond, that we live in a cage of thought from which there appears to be no escape. Thinking now dominates most people's lives to the exclusion of awareness of the emotions and instincts—the Ancestral Mind.

The Ancestral and Thinking Minds are based in different levels of the brain. There are three distinct levels in the development of the brain. The oldest part of the brain is the brain stem, on top of the spine at the base of the skull. This is called the *Reptilian Brain*, and it pre-dates human evolution. It's the seat of our instincts and deals with sensations and our immediate responses to them.

The next level surrounds this, and is about 50 million years old. This is the *Mammalian Brain*, which is the seat of our emotions. The Reptilian and Mammalian Brains form the Ancestral Mind.

The outer layers of the brain that surround both the Reptilian and Mammalian Brains form the cortex. Apparently the last six layers of this, called the *neo-cortex*, are the seat of the processes of thinking, abstract thought, planning and self-consciousness—the Thinking Mind.

With the neo-cortex's ability to create a sense of self-consciousness came a divergence between the Thinking Mind and the Ancestral Mind. Through being able to *speak about* our emotions instead of *being* them, and thus creating a sense of ourselves as separate from everything else, we began to perceive the world as linear, abstract and rational, and perceive past and future, with "me" in *here* and "everything else" out *there* to be acted upon.

Another thing that developed through the neo-cortex was the Thinking Mind's ability to respond to its own perceptions—to memory, abstract concepts and ideas about the future. This is the inner conversation that is now an integral part of everyone's life. This dialogue confirms our sense of self and is the basis for the emotional conflict we experience in life. Conflict arises because we usually don't distinguish between what has *actually* physically happened and what we *think* has happened. For our minds and bodies they are equally real.

Prior to the development of the neo-cortex, we had no sense of ourselves as separate—we lived our emotions and lived as an integral part of our environment. Our instincts were in-built ways to respond directly and reasonably accurately to the sensations we experienced. Emotions were a protective mechanism so we could learn and remember, fine-tune and create more flexibility in our responses. They also allowed us to communicate our internal states non-verbally.

In spite of the 20th century view of our unconscious minds as a sea of repressed and dangerous forces, our instincts and emotions are the source of all wisdom. They evolved to ensure the survival of our bodies by responding accurately to the world around us. *So emotions are still the way we keep in touch with what we need to know to survive.*

The three levels of the brain and Tantra
According to the meditation stream of Tantra, we experience the three levels of the brain through sensations focused at certain points in our bodies. The neo-cortex—thinking, planning, logic and inner conversations—we feel in our heads. In Tantra it's called the *head* or *crown centre*. In everyday conversation we say: "I've been planning things in my head; I've been working it out in my head; my head is full of ideas; I can't get that idea out of my head"; and so on. We also speak of being clear-headed and of having a head for certain things.

Our emotional life is centred in our hearts so this is where we experience the emotions and feelings of the Mammalian Brain. In Tantra this is called the *heart centre* and it's the centre of our emotional intelligence. In ordinary conversation we speak of being warm-hearted, of having a heart-to-heart conversation, of being broken-hearted when we feel intense emotional pain, of meeting at the heart, or being open-hearted.

We experience our instincts as sensations in our abdomen and this is the region of the Reptilian Brain. In Tantra this centre is called the *navel centre*. As we often refer to our instincts as "gut feelings", I like to call this centre the *gut*. A businessperson will make a crucial decision based on his or her "gut feeling" rather than the information at hand. We say we have had a gutful of something or someone when our territorial boundaries have been crossed. Someone either has the guts to do something or they don't. We are, in a very real sense, grounded in our gut.

So according to Tantra, we experience our Thinking Mind in our head and our Ancestral Mind in our body. Our head is the centre of clarity, discrimination, reason and logic—this is where we create divisions and define things. Our heart is the centre of warmth, emotional intelligence and the feeling of connection with everything. This is where we feel our equality and unity with everything that lives, and feel ourselves as an integral part of life and the universe. Our gut is the centre of direct response and action. It's where we experience the immediacy of life and our earthiness.

The monkey and the elephant

The meditation tradition has a classic image representing the two minds: a *monkey* (Thinking Mind) riding on the back of an *elephant* (Ancestral Mind). The monkey has a wonderful view—it can see clearly where it is going and where it has come from. Branches, fruit and nuts are in easy reach, so it jumps around, grabbing at whatever it can. It doesn't even know the elephant exists, let alone that it is riding on the elephant's back.

The elephant has no awareness of the monkey either. It can't see far ahead, and is only concerned with what is immediately in front of it and its immediate needs for survival, responding to its deep-seated instincts. It simply goes where it has been conditioned to go, lumbering along, slowly and inexorably. While the monkey is small and quick, the elephant is large and slow.

The monkey doesn't realise it is not deciding where it is going—it's literally being taken for a ride by the elephant. Because it can see, it has the illusion of making decisions, but it can't get anywhere without the elephant. *There could be no better representation of the Thinking Mind*.

Because the elephant carries the monkey, the monkey goes where the elephant goes. However, the elephant has nothing like the view of the monkey. It cannot plan or see the past and future. It is slow and powerful and motivated by its instincts. *This is the Ancestral Mind*.

This image demonstrates that the monkey is totally dependent on the elephant. The elephant could survive without the monkey, but the monkey is literally riding on the elephant's back. This explains why neat, well-planned decisions often have little relationship with what happens on the ground. For example, in universities and other institutions, decisions tend to be based on the belief that once the paper is written the job is done. But action is a different thing altogether—it is usually decided by instincts and emotions rather than what is written on paper.

When the Thinking Mind is slowed down and kept in touch with the body, so that plans are checked physically before being executed, the two can work together and the results can be extraordinary.

> My French piano teacher insisted I slow my practice down to the point where I became conscious of every tiny physical movement of my hands and fingers. No teacher had ever asked this before, and I found it very difficult to do—it took incredible patience. However, the results were miraculous because eventually the music became ingrained in my body and was effortless to play—it played itself. I was completely free from thinking about it, so I could let go and enjoy it and I never forgot it. Playing the piano became like riding a bike—it was there in my body.

So the moment of humility and awakening arises for the monkey when it sees the elephant. (In the stream of Insight meditation, insight refers to the moment of seeing the Ancestral Mind and seeing that the Thinking Mind is dependent on it.) They can then talk to each other, because the elephant decides where the action is, but can't see into the future. The monkey, with its clear view and ability to move quickly from one sense object to another, can gather information and plan ahead. The monkey can see the best place to go but the elephant has to take them there.

Two minds—two languages

The Thinking Mind, although it can use imagery, speaks mainly through the language of concepts, through words. Language came into being about 35000 years ago and written language is even younger—about 8000 years old. This means the Thinking Mind is a relative newcomer.

Images are the voice of the Ancestral Mind. When you are in an absorbed state of meditation, you will notice images arising; often fleeting, but sometimes clear to the point of seeming real. These hypnagogic images can also arise when you are just about to fall asleep, or have just woken up. They are an integral part of our dreams.

The Ancestral Mind can also think, but its thinking is not self-conscious or self-reflective. In other words, there is no sense of you thinking as there is with the Thinking Mind. Through its ability to hold a constant inner conversation, the Thinking Mind can completely dominate the Ancestral Mind, so we now live divorced from our instincts and emotions. The images through which they communicate are drowned out by the chatter in our heads.

Making contact with the body

Most people are awed by the peace and bliss they feel when they begin to make contact with their bodies through meditating. Then after a couple of classes, they become aware of how much traffic normally goes through their minds. They may then feel they are not doing well in their meditation, or even that they are losing the ability to do it. But in fact they have reached the first stage of meditation, where they are detached from the undercurrent of thought that usually runs our lives.

Many people then experience images from their Ancestral Mind as it now has space to be heard. Through meditation, you can open a new world as you discover that these images have a structure, and make as much sense as any other language—once you learn how to read it.

Your body communicates through images and feelings because the instincts and emotions of the older parts of the brain can only be felt in your body. Your relationship with your body becomes more intimate and fulfilling when you know how to listen to what it is saying. You feel *inside* your body instead of being a disembodied observer watching it from outside. You feel whole, connected and sane.

The world of the Ancestral Mind—images, symbols, dreams and the imagination—is what Carl Jung called the *collective unconscious*[17]. It was rediscovered in the 20th century, through Freud's use of dream analysis, and then through artists and poets, surrealists and symbolists. From the Thinking Mind's point of view it was unconscious, but it has *always been conscious* as far as our bodies are concerned.

Jung coined the term *collective unconscious* because he discovered that a great deal of imagery crossed time, cultures and races. He called such images archetypes and in meditation, when you access this level of imagery, images often appear in a particular order or in direct relation to things you are experiencing in your life. For example, you can see the stars, moon and sun and meet the earth mother, wise old man, imp, and friend who guide you.

Balancing the two minds

As we have seen, the cortex and neo-cortex rest on, and are supported by, the Mammalian and Reptilian Brains. In the same way, the Thinking Mind rests on, and is supported by, the Ancestral Mind. Tantric texts describe the mind as *riding on the energy winds and currents of the body*. This sounds arcane and esoteric but it means that our thoughts and emotions do not operate separately. If we are in a good state emotionally, then our thinking runs smoothly. If our emotions are running wild, then so will our thoughts.

When you feel the effect of emotions in the body, you discover that describing them as winds and currents isn't as strange as it sounds because this is exactly what they feel like—sometimes smooth and gentle; other times stormy and ferocious.

Although the Thinking Mind has been able to drown out the Ancestral Mind with its endless conversation, it cannot be divorced from it. The art of balance in meditation is to become aware of both of them, opening to the images and feelings of the Ancestral Mind, and noticing how our emotions affect the way we think. In this way you create a working partnership between the two minds, and so between your mind and body. Believing that one can or should dominate the other is a complete illusion, because it is impossible.

Recognising balance

In a sense, the two extremes of your mind are the Thinking Mind and the Ancestral Mind. Normally they are poles apart, so slewed towards thinking during the day that the Ancestral Mind is unconscious, then at night, while asleep, your mind swings to the opposite extreme so that the Thinking Mind is unconscious.

Meditation opens up the space in which both minds operate—that is, it reveals the context they live in and the foundation on which they both rest. This foundation is *fundamental awareness*—the state of infinite consciousness. When you meditate, you tap into this awareness, where nothing in particular is happening, but there are no boundaries and anything can happen. You might experience it as complete stillness, or a slightly floating feeling, as though you are resting in space.

Here you have equal access to both sides of your mind and the two languages of concepts and images. As you rest in the still space of fundamental awareness, you can be aware of thoughts, feelings, sensations and images as they come and go, without being caught in them, because you can just watch them in a detached way. You can see how the images of your mind relate to emotions and sensations in your body. You are aware of your *whole mind* as it rests in its natural state.

Chapter 20: A map of the mind

There are two major differences between Jung's map of the psyche and the meditation map of the mind, and these highlight the different orientations of Western and Eastern culture.

The map of the mind outlined in this chapter provides the structural basis for the philosophy and psychology of meditation. It comes from the Insight stream of the Buddhist meditation tradition and is based on the experience of seeing how the human mind actually works.

This map rests on an understanding of our mental processes which is very different from the way Western culture understands the human mind. Therefore, this chapter also briefly describes Jung's map of the psyche[18] to provide a Western perspective, which reveals how different its underlying assumptions are from the Eastern orientation, and how these assumptions pervade the way we see ourselves and the world around us.

A western map of the mind: the four functions

Perhaps the best known aspect of Carl Jung's work is his description of psychological types. This has formed the basis for popular psychological tests used in business, psychology, and major institutions. Jung described it as a map of the psyche, which he divided into four functions: **thinking, feeling, sensing** and **intuition**. These are "compass points" from which people orient themselves. Jung's thesis was that everyone uses one of these functions as their main point of reference and develops it accordingly, which determines their personality type.

For example, some people use thinking as their main reference point—they think about things before making decisions, weighing the pros and cons. Others might use feeling, and by this Jung meant the ability to judge or value things and situations as good or bad, useful or useless and so on. Some people orient themselves through their sensing, viewing the world according to the myriad details the senses provide; and others predominantly use their intuition, which gives them an overview of the world and situations they find themselves in.

Sensing and intuition are input functions—they provide the raw data the mind works with. Thinking and feeling are functions that organise the data provided by sensing and intuition, so everyone gains their information about the world predominantly through their sensing or intuition, and organises it through their thinking or feeling.

The map is polarised in the sense that you can't think *and* feel at the same time, and you can't use your sensing *and* your intuition at the same time. So people who develop one of these functions tend to repress the opposite function and it becomes what Jung called *the shadow*. When we say things like, "I'm not myself today" or "I was beside myself" we are experiencing our shadow side.

A good example of this is the joke, "My mind is made up, don't confuse me with facts", which is a typical feeling orientation to life. And the corollary is the typical attitude of the thinker who makes a decision according to the facts as they stand or the ideas presented on paper, and can't understand the fuss when people react unpredictably because the decision didn't take into account the feelings of those who would be affected by it.

The personality types Jung described are defined by the strongest function and this is usually supported by one other function. Here is the map of the thinking type.

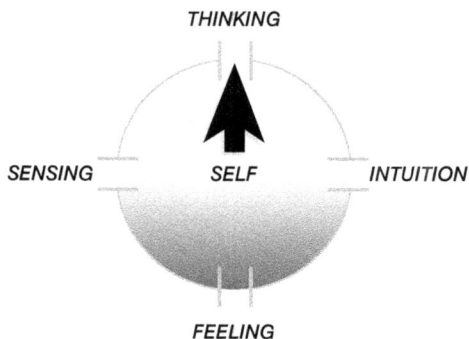

I've chosen thinking here because it is the dominant function of our culture. If we look at the map from this point of view, the self, in the centre of the map, is focused on thinking. It has access to sensing and intuition at the sides (almost like peripheral vision), so these can be its input functions. However, because of the self's orientation towards thinking, feeling is in the background—it is in the shadow. So feeling is the repressed and undeveloped function.

Usually only one of the other functions is developed strongly, for example sensing, so a person or culture might predominantly use thinking, backed up by sensing. Such a person or culture would still have access to the intuition, but in a weak form. To give you a feeling for a different orientation, Tibetan culture has intuition as its strong function, backed up by feeling (the second strongest function) with access to thinking, so sensing is in the shadow.

Here are some brief examples of the four different personality types from this map, to give you an idea of how it can be applied.

The sensing type
This type has developed their sensing function to a high degree; for example, a sportsperson, physiotherapist or mechanic, and supports this with thinking or feeling. They would have access to both but their intuition would be in the shadow.

The thinking type
An administrator, business person or philosopher has developed their thinking function and would support this with facts and detail (sensing) or with their gut feel for the big picture (intuition). Their feeling function would be in the shadow.

The feeling type
An artist, musician, society hostess or "people person" has strongly developed their feeling function. This means they orient themselves through their values—how they feel about things. They would support this with their sensing or intuition but their thinking function would be in the shadow.

The intuitive type
An entrepreneur or visionary has developed their intuition strongly and would support it with thinking or feeling, or have access to both at different times. Their sensing function would be in the shadow.

The Buddhist meditation tradition presents a map of the mind with five functions, which I call five stages in the process of consciousness. While Jung's map is based on the self, the Buddhist map of the mind goes beyond the self and outlines how consciousness actually works— this is a profoundly different orientation.

An eastern map of the mind: the process of consciousness
There are two major differences between the Buddhist meditation map and Jung's map of the psyche, and these highlight the different

orientations of Western and Eastern culture. Firstly, the meditation map of the mind includes the body whereas Jung's map is bodiless (as all traditional Western maps and theories about the mind or psyche have tended to be).

Secondly, Jung's map is focused on the self, whereas the meditation map doesn't even consider the self—it just examines how *consciousness* works. In our culture, when we speak of consciousness we mean the process by which we become aware of things, so we see consciousness in terms of *us* being aware of something that is *not us*. However, in meditation this is only one form of consciousness, called *self-referencing* consciousness.

The meditation map outlines the *process* of self-referencing consciousness, but not from an individual point of view. This is a profound difference. Because Jung worked in a culture that views consciousness as *self-consciousness* he assumed that everything we experience is orientated from an individual point of view. From this perspective, everything is seen in straight lines with a positive and negative pole, which sets up opposites—a strong function and a shadow function.

The meditation map of the mind offers a completely different way of orienting ourselves. If consciousness is a process, and self-consciousness is only one aspect of this process, it means there is a way to view and experience consciousness outside our normal orientation. Here, consciousness is not personal or fixed in a particular direction and this provides many more options than with the self always being at the centre.

The two ways of seeing—focused and open

From a self-referencing point of view we can only see in straight lines—we are here, something else is there, and we can either move towards it or away from it. We see ourselves in a story or narrative—those who are moving in the same direction are friends, those going in a different direction are neutral, and those moving in the opposite direction are enemies.

When we set goals we tend to see ourselves as small moving towards a bigger self, progressing and developing, increasing our power, money, number of friends and so on. This is a dynamic and useful way to see ourselves and our lives, but the cost is that we ignore a lot of what is happening. For example, we can't get a clear view of the environment we are operating in or our relationship with it and we take for granted the people and things supporting us. We also don't see what doesn't fall into our line of view—we ignore the whole context of life itself.

The meditation map of the mind offers a much broader perspective. For example, the self, as self-referencing consciousness, simply becomes a point of view. The self itself is a reference point; it is the thought, feeling, idea or image that allows us to compare what we are viewing with what we already know—the narrative that makes up our memory.

Therefore, the self is not seen as fixed, permanent or stable, but as constantly changing, depending on the situation we are in. For example, when you compare yourself at the beach with how you are at work, you'll see they are two different people.

Another way to understand this is to visualise the Western perspective as a straight line, and the Eastern perspective as a circle. A straight line has a beginning and an end, and is moving in a particular direction; it is focused. A circle is not going anywhere—it has no direction and is timeless, so *everything* is in view, as with peripheral vision. Here you are not focused on anything in particular so everything is open. You can choose what to focus on at any particular time.

These two ways of thinking and experiencing derive from the two distinct ways the mind can operate. The mind has the ability to reference and compare things, moving from one point to another, and seeing things in terms of cause and effect. It also has the ability to move beyond space and time by becoming completely still, so it can open to the immediate moment fully, or to the big picture.

Self-referencing is dynamic, and the Western perspective reflects this in that invariably we see our minds only as thoughts—we don't see that our mind can also be still. When you are absorbed, your mind and body are balanced and still. This is a more fundamental state than thinking, and here you have access to all the mind's processes. When the mind is not focused on anything in particular, it is like an engine in neutral. You have the time and space to look at the whole engine because it is not being used to perform a particular task.

Understanding the mind in this way enormously supports a calm state in meditation. It frees you from having to always see yourself in reference to everyone and everything in your life. You have the option of simply *being* and *seeing*, rather than always *going somewhere* and *doing something*. Your view of yourself and the world can become deeper, richer and more flexible because you can *see* the processes of your mind, instead of being caught in them.

The five steps in the process of consciousness

The meditation map of the mind outlines how we become aware of objects when they interact with our senses. The five steps in this process of consciousness are:

1. **The physical body**—your body and senses
2. **Sensation**—what you feel when you sense something
3. **Perception**—your ability to name and identify things
4. **Narration**—the memories, stories and tendencies which shape your decisions
5. **Consciousness**—the quality of awareness itself

Note that this model includes the physical aspect of the mind—the body and senses—and consciousness itself. Although Jung's map of the psyche does include sensing, it is a mental process, one step removed from the actual physical reality of the body (i.e. the senses themselves). This is an important distinction, because the meditation map doesn't divorce the body from the mind; it includes it as an integral part of the process of consciousness. Without a body there are no senses, and without senses there are no sensations. The meditation map of the mind is presented below.

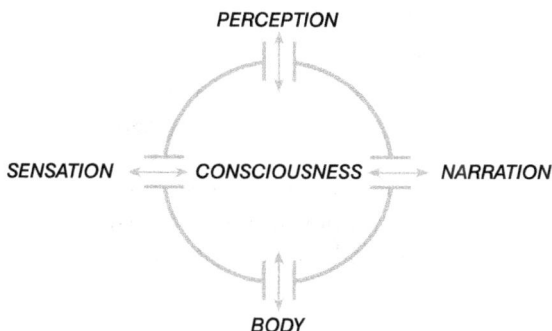

PERCEPTION

SENSATION ← → CONSCIOUSNESS ← → NARRATION

BODY

Placing consciousness (the light of awareness) in the centre instead of the self completely changes the emphasis and feeling because the map is much more open—there is a sense of space when the centre is not fixed and limited.

Let's compare the two maps. Imagine yourself in the centre of a room with four windows—one in front of you, one on your left, another on your right and one behind you. In Jung's map you can see clearly out of the window in front of you, a little out of the side windows and nothing behind you. Behind you is a world you can feel but never see, so it is dark and unknown (the shadow). This provides a sense of the Western view of the mind. It illustrates exactly what happens when you focus on a goal, and when you are moving in a certain direction—just like driving a car.

Now imagine yourself being free to move around and look through any of the windows. You can also look around the room and see every part of it clearly—it is all light so nothing is dark or unknown. If you were in a car, the only time you could do this is when the car is still—when you are not going anywhere. This gives an immediate feeling for the difference between the two maps.

In the meditation map, the self, instead of being a fixed entity at the centre of the mind, can be identified with any one of the steps in the process of consciousness. For example, some people identify with their bodies; others with the sensations they feel; some with the way they perceive and name what they experience; others with deciding which story will dominate or with creating the stories; and finally, some identify with consciousness itself—with seeing and knowing. This map includes the self in all its variations, but also *everything* you experience.

The Three C Technique is a practical way to apply the meditation map of the mind to your daily life.

The Three C Technique

From this map you can also begin to understand how the Three C Technique works. When you **Catch the moment** you realise that you are beginning to act in a habitual way. So, you **Clear the space** by doing a meditation to allow your mind to become still. You move from placing yourself at the centre of your mind to allowing an open state of awareness to take central place. Your mind is calm, clear and open and you are free from the way you habitually see yourself.

This means that you shift from being able to see in one direction only, which is your usual, fixed point of view, to being open to points of view you would normally not be aware of. In this moment you have a choice because you become aware of your perceptions—how you are seeing things—the sensations in your body, and what your body itself it actually doing, instead of being locked into the memories, stories, emotions and habits that you would normally be focused on.

> A simple example of this process in my own life has been my relationship with chocolate—as soon as I felt lacking in energy, I would hit the chocolate. The first couple of pieces would taste excellent and feel fine, but of course I would keep eating it.
>
> I decided that as we all need one compulsion in our lives, chocolate was a relatively harmless one. However, one day while having a chocolate binge, instead of my mind automatically jumping into the stories and pleasant associations I had with chocolate, I created the space to actually feel what my body was experiencing in the present. The sensation was right there in my awareness—and after the initial taste, it was not pleasant. After this, chocolate stopped being an obsession.

Using meditation to open up this moment in the process of consciousness enables you to **Change the habit**. All experience exists only in the present. We can either allow ourselves to open to the direct sensory experience of our bodies *or* allow our lives to be dominated by our memories and expectations. Our minds can't be focused on both simultaneously.

The difference between sensations and emotions

The meditation map of the mind makes a clear distinction between sensations and emotions, whereas Western culture tends to run them together. Because we *feel* both sensations and emotions inside our bodies, we tend to believe they are an integral part of who we are.

As your meditation practice develops, and you become aware of what you are feeling instead of being caught in it, you come to understand the difference between sensations and emotions. Sensations are the immediate response of our bodies to what happens—pleasant, painful or neutral. Emotions are the feelings associated with the memories and stories (narratives) we have built up over time. *Every* memory and story has an emotion associated with it, so emotions are also associated with our thinking. Sensations are generated by what is actually happening; emotions are generated by what we *think* and *remember* about what is happening.

Being open to your sensations

Your body is sensing all the time and the sensations you experience are your immediate contact with your body. They are also your direct experience of everything that happens in your life, so you can keep your thoughts and emotions in their proper place by being open to your sensations. It's rather sad that we spend so much time trying to escape them.

Many people are afraid of their sensations because they feel they are not in control of them. Meditation provides the resources and confidence to stay with a sensation because you can step back from any thought or emotion. By meditating you literally dissolve the stories, emotions and habits and return to a balanced state where you can just watch sensations *without getting caught in emotions*.

Breathing meditation is particularly useful because every thought, emotion, state of mind and sensation has a breathing pattern. As they are working together all the time and have an immediate effect on each other, you can consciously intervene by concentrating on your breathing and bringing it to a slower, smoother rhythm, which will change the state you are experiencing.

Being afraid of bliss

Surprisingly, many people are also afraid of blissful sensations in their bodies. This fear can arise through what they have been taught, and from the fact that these sensations can't be controlled.

A teenage girl with an eating disorder who had attempted suicide was referred to me to learn meditation. She told me about an incident that had occurred a few years earlier, which had caused her to fear and distrust her sexuality. She took to meditating well and began to feel much more comfortable in her body. During our last session I received a shy, very sweet smile so I said, "Do you know that you are a very attractive young woman?" Her response was an immediate, confident look, straight into my eyes. We shared a hug as that was the end of our sessions. Her father was delighted at how she had managed to transform herself.

Another young man in his early twenties was referred to me by a psychologist who guessed that his fear of sensations was at the root of his problem. He suffered from a permanent skin rash on his hands, and had tried everything the medical profession had to offer. His relationship with his girlfriend had never been comfortable.

He loved drawing, so I asked to see his pictures, and they were rampantly sexual. He came from a repressive religious background and had no way to reconcile what he was actually sensing with what he had been taught. I was thankful that he had hung in there with the conflict he was experiencing. Learning meditation and being with someone who accepted what he was feeling gave him the calm to begin to open to his sensations. The rash was gone within three sessions and his relationship with his girlfriend flourished.

The power of meditation

The power of meditation lies in its ability to cut through the automatic process of consciousness and bring the mind's focus immediately and directly to the body. I believe that nearly all psychological disorders arise from narratives not being in accord with what is being felt. In other words, the mind, being focused on a thought or memory, has not properly registered the sensation of the body, so the two are in conflict.

Physically stored unpleasant memories can contaminate your future experience for minutes or hours. We all know what it's like to "get out of bed on the wrong side". People who suffer from depression have unconsciously mastered the ability to maintain their reaction to these kinds of memories for long periods. Others have mastered the ability to change emotional states at will, creating emotional freedom. The universe may deal a mixed hand of cards, but we can choose how and when to play them.

Meditation calms your body and emotions and creates space in your mind, returning your mind to its natural state of awareness. This immediately clears your mind of all thoughts and emotions—just for a second. In catching this moment it is possible to completely rebuild a circuit that might have been operating in a faulty way for years.

For example, in my obsession with chocolate, my story had overridden what my body was actually experiencing. Once I cleared my mind of the story, I could then accept the sensations in my body and name them according to what I was actually feeling instead of what had been imposed. The thoughts and emotions that accompanied the sensation were then appropriate, rather than in conflict with the experience of my body. I still like chocolate of course, but there's no longer a need to binge.

The next chapter describes three personality types, which the meditation tradition classifies according to the automatic, habitual response people have to an object.

Chapter 21: The three personality types— moving toward, stepping back and staying still

When faced with an object there are three ways you can react to it. You might be immediately attracted and move towards it, you might reject it outright and step back or you might not know what to do, so stay still.

Different meditations suit different people and the meditation tradition used a system of typing to determine this. The typology is based on how a person immediately, habitually reacts to a particular object, which determines their personality type.

There are three ways you can react to an object. You might be immediately attracted to it—curious and wanting to **move toward** it. This would lead to being open and generous or wanting to possess it and make it your own.

Another way to react would be to reject it outright or **step back** and keep your distance. You would want to examine it carefully before deciding whether to engage with it.

Another way to react would be **staying still**, not knowing whether to move forwards or backwards. You might be unable to decide how to respond because you could both want it and not want it simultaneously. So you would end up confused and become immobilised.

This typology is a simple but profound way to understand human behaviour. If you observe your own behaviour you will find that you have an immediate, habitual way of approaching people and the things and situations that come your way.

Each of the personality types has a positive and a negative aspect. When you **move towards** something you are very focused on what you want to achieve, but you are not looking at where you are coming from, the expectations you are bringing or whether the situation is sustainable. You completely ignore anything that might get in the way or bring unexpected consequences.

When **stepping back**, you are very clear about what you are moving away from, but not really looking at what you are getting yourself into. *From the frying pan into the fire* describes this very well.

And when you **stay still** you can see all the possibilities in any situation, but it can be very paralysing when it comes to making decisions. You end up being unable to move because if you do, you have to give up the options—you can't have it all.

Let's explore these types in more detail.

The positive aspects of the types

Moving toward—generosity

Curiosity is an extremely healthy form of desire. Nobody could survive without desire—you simply wouldn't eat or look after your body if it wasn't there. Being open to what is around you, questioning, keeping your senses open, wanting to know and understand, to see, hear, smell, taste and touch, engages you with life and other people.

When you are open and curious, wanting to get involved and engage with what is happening, you move forward, and in doing this you give yourself to the person or situation you are moving towards. This act of giving yourself is also an act of confidence—a powerful force that takes you beyond your perceived limitations and opens up strengths and possibilities you never knew you were capable of. It moves you, so that you experience what is meant by the Zen saying: *the action does itself rather than you doing it.* This is what it feels like when you give yourself and your energy completely to something.

I experienced this every time I walked onto a concert platform, as does every performer, because you have done all the technical work and all that is left is confidence. You just go out and let the concert take you over.

Stepping back—love

Desire is balanced by not rushing in where angels fear to tread. Being able to step back from a situation and question it is essential for a healthy life. Allowing time to come to know something or someone before engaging with them is a valuable old-fashioned quality that is gradually being lost.

In rushing headlong into a situation or a relationship, no matter how much confidence we might have or how much we want to give, we are not really looking at what it entails, what our expectations are or whether it is sustainable. Stepping back and giving yourself and the other person some space, enables you to move beyond your ideas and expectations about what you want to happen. This allows room for the relationship to grow because it takes into account the reality of what you are engaging with.

This is the way to love. Instead of assuming you know who someone is, and expecting them to behave in a certain way, you allow time to come to know each other. Politeness is a form of keeping your distance until you're sure that you really *are* prepared to engage, to pay the price and invest the time, and by doing this, the move forward can be committed and full-hearted. Or, you can disengage with no harm done. In doing this you are being kind to others and respectful of their feelings. The preparedness to show this respect is the foundation of love. The well-known teacher Krishnamurti[19] used to say that *the way to come to love is by discarding the known*.

Allowing time for the preliminaries with people and situations is a true sign of respect. Australians, with our rather casual approach to each other, can get frustrated when entering the social rituals of Asian cultures. It seems a lot of time is being wasted instead of just getting down to the business at hand. But social rituals enable you to take your time testing someone, coming to know them, seeing if you can trust and work with them. Rushing into deals and becoming hypnotised by stories of what can be achieved, instead of looking carefully at the people involved, can mean a lot of time and expense in the painful process of getting out later.

I was struck by the cultural differences I encountered as a student in France. It suited my personality, and I could never understand why many people found the French impolite. They were extraordinarily polite, and insisted on all the preliminary rituals before entering any relationship—for example, even if you went into a shop to buy something. They took pride in their shop and what they produced, and you were expected to respect this. If you did the relationship became very warm. There was an expectation of courtship which is rather foreign to us.

In Australia, if people are asked to do something, the first response is usually, "Yeah, not a problem". But if it gets a bit difficult, the interest can wane. In France, if you asked if something could be done, the answer was invariably "Non monsieur, that is not possible". However, if you were prepared to be patient and follow the rituals you found that suddenly there would be a real commitment to getting it done.

Another side to love is the passion to change something unjust or destructive. This personality type will engage with total commitment to create fairness and equality in the cause of social justice. And they are the people who fight to protect the environment against the destruction that accompanies rampant consumerism.

Staying still—wisdom

Being able to see both sides of a situation, the cost and the benefit, is a valuable life skill. It's a combination of curiosity and scepticism that opens up the whole picture and enables you to see all the options in any situation. It can lead to lateral thinking and to a unique and creative way of responding.

The ability to do this is the foundation of wisdom. Wisdom comes from the Latin word, *video*, which means "to see". So wisdom is the ability to *see clearly* the whole situation. However, this requires being still, which is why all meditation begins with learning to be still.

It's not always an easy thing to do. We are so driven by thoughts and emotions that we find it hard to stop, so our lives become increasingly busy. But the more we move, the less we can see clearly. Only by staying still can you become aware of what your body is telling you. You are open to the experience of your senses, so are seeing, fully and directly, what you are *experiencing*, rather than filtering it through stories.

The negative aspects of the types

Let's look at the negative aspects. Anyone advising on the stock market knows that greed and fear are the forces driving it. In a nutshell, these are the two negative aspects of moving toward something and stepping back from it.

Moving forward—greed

Interest and curiosity can tip over into obsession, and then moving forward, achieving goals, making things your own, and winning at all costs, if unchecked and unbalanced, become outright greed. This is the insatiable desire to possess everything that comes your way. No matter how much you own, the bottom line always changes, and more is never enough.

Stepping back—anger

Stepping back from something to take stock can lead, as your mind fixes on it and you lose your emotional balance, to becoming suspicious and fearful of it. This leads to wanting to get rid of it at all costs, and eventually to anger.

The interesting thing about anger or even its extreme form, hatred, is that you can't be indifferent toward the object of your anger. You really care about it; this is why it is the other side of love. We get very angry with things that don't turn out as we want, and this often means we had an expectation about how it would turn out.

When we are angry and attempt to reject something, we stop looking at it, and are not prepared to learn what our expectations actually were—what it was we didn't see about it. So we can get into fights over things we feel have happened, whether they have or not, and to rejecting things, people and situations because we are afraid of being rejected ourselves.

To withdraw from a situation or person you need to have accepted what is happening to see it clearly and then make a decision to withdraw. If we reject without seeing what is happening we often run into the same situation all over again.

Staying still—confusion

Confusion arises when, instead of seeing clearly what is in front of us, we get so overwhelmed by information and possibilities, by not coping and fear, that we stop seeing altogether. Everything turns into a blur and we find it impossible to make a decision, let alone act in a definite way.

Confusion is the other side of wisdom because it arises when you are aware, in a subconscious way, of all the possibilities in front of you, and find them overwhelming. You then can't make decisions or move—it's a form of emotional paralysis.

The three types in summary

These personality types are based on the fact that when two things come into contact they can be attracted to each other, repelled from each other or held in suspension. With human beings this involves our emotions, so each of these movements is accompanied by a particular emotion.

When **moving towards** something we experience *desire*. This can be healthy and when it is we move towards someone or something in a completely open state, giving ourselves to the person or situation. Healthy desire is based on genuine need—our own or someone else's. It's a state of honesty where what you see is what you get. It's refreshing and energising.

When desire is unhealthy the move is not straightforward. You are more focused on calculating, "What can I get out of it?" or "What's in it for me?" than on the person or situation in front of you. This will inevitably create a backlash as the reality of the object or person is asserted, which will eventually create conflict.

When **moving away** from something or someone we experience *caution*. This can be healthy when we allow space for the person or situation to reveal themselves and enter a dialogue to find out what is, or isn't, possible. It becomes unhealthy when we reject something or someone outright rather than being open to who they are.

And in **standing still** we keep our *balance*. This is healthy when we use it to examine what we are faced with. We weigh the options, costs and benefits, take into account the context and environment and the impact it is likely to have—and then act accordingly. It becomes unhealthy when we are overwhelmed by what we see and allow the mind to fuse—we become confused and incapable of seeing clearly what we are dealing with.

Most of what each personality type does falls within the spectrum between the two extremes summarised.

The next chapter describes the different meditation objects, which are variously suited to these different personality types.

Chapter 22: The different meditation objects

There was never any rule that one meditation suits all, or even that a particular meditation was suitable for all occasions.

Different meditations were designed for different purposes, for different personality types, and to take you to different levels of absorption. A well qualified meditation teacher should be able to guide someone to quickly find what kinds of meditation suit and work well for them.

Although Buddhism outlines forty different meditation objects, a number of them are impossible to do today—unless you are a mortician or do autopsies! Ten are based on following the different stages of decomposition of a corpse.

This chapter outlines a broad selection of meditation objects; there are meditations using physical objects, contemplations, meditations on light and space, states of love, and analytical meditations. There are also meditations on the infinite states of absorption.

Each meditation will take you to a different level of concentration or absorption and different meditations are also particularly well suited to the different personality types discussed in Chapter 21. To refresh your memory, these types are based on the immediate, habitual reaction people have to an object. They could find it attractive (**moving forward**), be wary of it (**stepping back**), or not know how to respond (**staying still**). At the end of the chapter you will find a quick reference chart to match the meditation to level of concentration or absorption and personality type.

The meditation objects

The first four meditation objects we will look at are the four physical elements: earth, water, fire and air (or wind).

Earth, water, fire, air

These meditations can make you more acutely aware of the world around you, and of the feeling response they evoke in your body—more connected, vital and alive.

There are detailed instructions in the texts about how to set these up for meditation but I have found that the following ways are very effective.

Earth

To meditate on earth, fill a plain bowl with sand, clay or soil. The earth needs to be clean and fine enough that you can make the surface smooth. The recommended size is around 25cm—it needs to be large enough to hold your attention without being too close.

Another way to meditate on earth is to find a clean rock that attracts you, about the size of your hand. Large quartz crystals are inexpensive and easy to obtain. A ploughed field, long beach, cliff face or Zen rock garden are also very effective for meditating on the earth.

Water

To meditate on water, simply fill a plain, preferably white bowl with water.

You can also informally meditate on a lake or sea. Who hasn't sat beside water and just relaxed? What makes it meditation is becoming conscious of what you are doing and feeling the effect of it in your body.

Meditating on a wild, stormy sea is an exhilarating experience. Waves crashing on rocks and spray soaring into the air give a thrill right through the body as you open to the power and energy of the sea.

Fire

The classical way to meditate on fire is to use a candle; focus on the place where the flame splits.

People instinctively meditate on fire when they go camping. Allowing your mind to rest on the flames of an open fire—or a fire in a combustion heater—becomes a perfect meditation.

Air

To meditate on air, let your mind gently rest on grass moving in the wind. Opening your mind to the sound of the grass or trees moving in a gentle wind is another effective way to meditate on air. Feeling the movement of the air on your skin, opening to the sensation of being caressed by the air, is a wonderful experience.

Colours

Four colours were classically given as meditation objects: yellow, white, red and blue. I like to add green to the list. Traditionally, yellow is associated with earth, white with water, red with fire and blue with air or space.

Yellow speeds up the mind and opens it, loosening it. Red also speeds up the mind but concentrates it, tightening it. Blue slows down the mind and opens and loosens it. Green also slows down the mind but concentrates and tightens it. We instinctively experience the effects of these colours in that yellow and red are energising and blue and green are calming. (Pay attention to the colours used in packaging on the supermarket shelves—yellow and red predominate to catch your attention; blue and green are used for environmentally-friendly products.)

White can be both colourless and all colours so in meditation it is used to stimulate clarity—opening the mind to the experience of the fundamental state of awareness which is clear, open and spacious. In meditation, blue is used to calm the mind and green to relax the body.

To meditate on colour:

Cut a round disc, about 20–25cm in diameter, from a coloured sheet, or colour in a disc of thick white paper or cardboard. Ensure the colour is thick and even (oil-based pastels from the supermarket work well).

Rest your eyes in the centre of the disc, then close them occasionally to absorb the colour and see if you can visualise it (you might see the complementary colour). As you develop this meditation, aim to see exactly the same colour with your eyes closed as when they are open, so your mental image and the object are the same.

As you meditate on the different colours, explore the effect they have on your body and feelings.

Compare the effect when you move from one colour to another.

You can also use flowers or gem stones as meditation objects of colour. For green you can use leaves from a tree or bird feathers.

Informal meditations on colour can be done any time you are outside, either as a quick Spot Meditation to open your senses, or as a longer meditation to let your mind rest in a particular colour. Watching the colours at sunset and sunrise creates time for refreshing and nourishing your inner life.

Space

See Chapter 15, which outlines both formal and informal meditations on space.

Light and consciousness

Light and consciousness have always been linked in the meditation tradition. As formal objects of meditation, they are considered the same—when you meditate on light, your mind also opens to the experience of consciousness.

> Let your mind rest on the light reflected on the leaves of trees, or on sunlight or moonlight reflected on water.
>
> Become aware of a feeling or image of the light filling your body; you may even reach a stage where your entire body is shimmering light.

Meditating on death

Death has become a major taboo in our culture, to the extent that doctors feel they have failed when a patient dies, and actually say they "lost" the patient or couldn't "save" her. Death is never discussed and death and dying are hidden from the public view, so we are unprepared for facing death. In the meditation tradition death was a form of meditation—both the physical reality and contemplating the idea of death.

> In India over two millenia ago, bodies were simply left to decay and disintegrate in the charnel ground. During my first visit to Calcutta I saw a woman dying in the street—I was in my early thirties, and the physical shock of this experience was enormous. Although I had accepted the reality of death in my meditation work, this was an immediate, physical blow to the senses which spoke directly to my body. She and I were intimately joined by this common destiny.
>
> I also remember riding my motorbike home from university one night, and seeing a cat that had been run over. I stopped and went over to find that it was still alive, so I picked it up and took it into a nearby park to sit with it as it died. The cat accepted me picking it up without any distress, and after I placed it on the ground it lay for about ten minutes breathing quietly and then died peacefully.
>
> Of course, death is not always peaceful. It can be violent, prolonged and painful. However, with meditation, people can build resources of emotional calm and concentration which enables them to face the reality of death. They do not have to

maintain the defence of ignoring it, but can become aware of this part of life so they can deal with pain, their own death and the death of loved ones, in a way that strengthens inner resources and a sense of compassion.

Two of my students died of cancer in their fifties. One contracted it suddenly and the other had been expected to die in his thirties but kept himself alive for over seventeen years by building up his own resources, including meditation. The former, while in hospice facing his death, told me that it was only through this experience that he came to truly understand the ideas and experiences he had been introduced to through meditation, and how they could be used.

The other student refused to take drugs because he preferred to feel the reality of the pain. When it became evident he could no longer survive the disease, and was about to be moved to a hospice, he simply let go and died the day he was to be moved. Both men died peacefully and I developed an enormous respect and love for them, and felt privileged to share their experiences.

Meditating on death is a way to accept the earthiness of our bodies and lives. It takes you directly beyond all the ideas and fears around death to its physical reality so you can watch it without prejudices. Without death, life would be absolutely impossible.

Begin with something easily accessible like a dead leaf or flower. Normally these things are thrown out when they are dead, but you can keep them a while longer and use them as a meditation object.

Contemplations
Like all forms of contemplation, these meditations are reflections on ideas, qualities and states of mind that help keep your mind and emotions in a healthy, balanced state.

The body
Because it's so easy to become lost in ideas, this contemplation brings you back to the reality of your body.

Simply use the word **BODY** to keep bringing your mind back.

The word *body* is related to the Buddhist word *Bodhi*, which means to be awake and understand. Its root meaning is "to bud", or "to open up", so it includes the idea of the senses being open and wide awake.

By contemplating the body we can feel its limits—the physical boundary to life that gives us clear definition, sharpness and direction. This opens us to life so that we stay aware of how vivid our senses are and how precious our bodies are. It's the fact that our bodies are constantly changing; and have a beginning and an end, that make them so precious.

Coming to know the body through anatomy books is another way to contemplate the human body. This can be a good antidote to idealising the body and trying to make it perfect, or to denigrating it. Looking at photographs of the internal world of the body can open your mind to a sense of awe at how this unbelievably intricate, delicate organism can exist at all.

> When you do a Bodyscan or the Mind and Body Washing Meditation (see Chapter 4) take a little longer to meditate on the different parts of your body.
>
> Try to visualise, or get a feeling for, the skeleton, nervous system, lymphatic system, heart, blood system, all the organs, muscles and tissues, the senses and the skin.

Death

Don Juan, the South American Indian shaman featured in Castaneda's popular books in the sixties, said to Castaneda that it was important to *let death sit on your left shoulder*. Reminding yourself of the reality of death encourages you to stay alert and use every moment of life. It's worth thinking about the idea that perhaps people aren't so much afraid of death as of *facing the fact they never lived their life fully*.

> Simply use the word **DEATH** to keep this reality in your mind.

Only through ignoring death and the limits of the body do people become destructive to themselves and the world, because their minds are not focused on reality but on their ideas and beliefs.

Openness

Allowing yourself to be open—to yourself, others and the life around you—balances the tendency we have to close ourselves up and remain concerned with our immediate self-interest. All unhealthy states of mind have an undercurrent of fear in them because looking out for number one is a rather anxious business—you always have to be on guard.

Openness means respecting yourself, and then respecting others. It's a form of active listening—being prepared to listen to your own body and to what others are saying. Sharing your life with others is a direct act of generosity, because it opens communication. When you are prepared to really see someone, listen to what they are saying and feel what their bodies are communicating, you are giving yourself to them. This is a practical way to free yourself from fear and it builds a real sense of confidence.

Repeating a mantra is an excellent way to open yourself; it clears the mind of its closed-circuit conversations, and allows you to listen with your body and heart.

> The mantra **OM MANI PADME HUM** is designed to keep you in touch with your heart and be completely open to others.
>
> You can also use a short phrase like **BE OPEN**, or single words like **LISTEN** or **OPENNESS**.

Peace

Being at peace with yourself is a wonderful thing; it comes from being able to accept everything about yourself and your life. This is not easy, but it's important to realise that until something is accepted it can't be seen—it's being ignored or repressed.

Meditation provides the ability to create and sustain the foundation of calm that allows things we normally couldn't cope with into our awareness. When you are balanced, you can watch the emotions and states of mind which dominate your life when we say "I've lost control" or "I've lost the plot".

In meditation, ignored or repressed emotions can move through your body instead of being stuck. A lot of meditation work involves mental and emotional "washing"—letting go of the waste that builds up in the system.

Peace is the result of accepting this process and being able to accept ourselves as we are. We can then extend this to other people and eventually to the world. Acceptance is not indifference in the sense of, "This is the way things are and they'll never change", but being prepared to *see things as they are.*

> Simply use the word **PEACE**, and allow a feeling of peace to expand through your body. If you wish, you can focus on different parts of your body as you do this.

Foundation of the mind

This contemplation reminds you that your thoughts are not your whole mind. The foundation of the mind is still, open and luminous, like the sky. Every thought or emotion you experience—ecstatic or agonising—will eventually return to this state. This is *the core or depth of your being*. Other names include *the ground of being* or the *natural mind*. Buddhists call it *Buddha nature*, and Christians may call it *God*.

> You can use words like **SPACE, LOVE, TRUTH** and **STILLNESS** to contemplate the foundation of your mind.

Before I learned meditation I touched on this experience—a deep sense of space in which everything rested—without knowing what it was. I called it *Love*, because in this state I felt a deep sense of connection with all of life.

Visualisation

Everything we see, we can only see because it reflects light. So light and form enable the eye and brain to distinguish physical objects. When we visualise things internally, we experience them in the same way—as light and form. However, because there is no physical object reflecting the light, they are forms of consciousness itself. This is why light and consciousness are considered synonymous in the meditation tradition.

When you visualise something it is therefore an aspect of *consciousness*—you are actually seeing an aspect of your mind. You can begin to understand all the different aspects of your mind—all the different qualities of consciousness—through visualisations that tap these different qualities.

In the Eastern tradition this is done by personifying each aspect, so the meditation tradition calls these visualisations "beings of light". For example, love has both female and male forms, and can be kind and peaceful, compassionate, ecstatic, sexual, or fierce (warning you where the boundaries are). However, because these come with the forms, structures and concepts of mediaeval, feudal societies, they don't always work well for us. Images from the incredibly old and rich landscape of Australia serve just as well to tap the different aspects of the mind.

There are images in nature that are still and peaceful; nurturing, safe and protective; images that are ancient and resonate with timelessness; images that are fiery and passionate, and others full of the power of nature at its wildest. All these qualities exist in our minds. Refer back to Chapter 4 for meditations using visualisation.

Breathing

Focusing on the breath is the simplest meditation in the tradition.

In the ancient languages of our culture, Greek and Latin, the words for *breath* also meant spirit. The Greek word for breath was *pneuma* and it survives in English as *pneumatic*, as in a pneumatic tyre (a tyre filled with air). In Latin the word was *spiritus* and, like *pneuma* it meant both breath and spirit. This is where the English word *spirit* comes from.

Pranayama exercises which control the breath form an important part of yoga. One meaning of the Sanskrit word *prana* is breath and its similarity with the Greek *pneuma* is striking. So breath and spirit were considered to be the same—breath was the spirit of life. In Tantric meditations you learn how to tap this spirit and feed your energies by directing your breath. This is invaluable for many health professionals who are literally drained of emotional energy.

With breathing meditations you can consciously create good feelings in your body. In fact, the whole repertoire of pleasure, both physical and emotional, is accessible when you know how to use your breath. It has the power to calm the mind to the point of stillness, heal both mind and body, create bliss in the body, and open up the whole mind.

Many students have come to major insights and decisions through meditating on the breath. People suffering from stress, anxiety, depression, and chronic pain, have either been cured and given up drugs, or learned to manage their lives much more successfully by learning how to use their breath. One young woman who had suffered from panic attacks for years, completely freed herself from them in one session of learning to meditate on the breath.

Refer back to Chapter 4 for a range of meditations using the breath.

Four boundless states of mind—the states of love

Meditating on love is common to both the Western and Eastern traditions. In Chapter 17 I referred to a textbook called *The Cloud of Unknowing* written by an anonymous Western monk for his students in the 13th century[20]. This book aimed to lead students to a point where they could let go to enter a state of unknowing, and penetrate it to reach a state of union. While consciously following the breath, the student was asked to use the word "God" on the in-breath and "love" on the out-breath—they filled themselves with the love of God and breathed it out to the world. A Tibetan exercise asks you to have the courage to breathe in the pain of someone else and then transform it by breathing out love.

In the group of meditations on boundless states of mind, two of them are familiar to us as states of love: they are **kindness** and **compassion**. The other two, **sharing joy** and a state of balance or **equanimity**, we don't always associate with love.

However, sharing a person's pain is viewed as an act of love, so why not sharing someone else's joy? It's a wonderful thing to do. And keeping yourself emotionally balanced (*equanimity*) in the face of everything we experience with other people is the foundation of being able to be open and respect their feelings and experiences.

These meditations are called boundless states because they are designed to take you beyond the boundaries of your view of yourself and your world. They become increasingly inclusive, until you can hold in your mind people, places and other forms of life way beyond your immediate experience, and consciously create feelings of acceptance, warmth, understanding, compassion and joy. In this way you are opening yourself to states of mind and feelings without any boundaries, and strengthening yourself emotionally.

Kindness

The first boundless state is a feeling of open-hearted kindness, toward yourself and others. *Kindness* is based on the word *kin* so a meditation on kindness brings to mind our kinship with everything that lives—that we're all in it together.

Kindness is a state of being. It's the simple acceptance of the fact that our bodies all live within the same limits, that we are totally dependent on the earth for our survival, and that all other people and life forms share this with us. You view yourself and the world from the heart, opening to a feeling of kinship with all of life.

In contemplating kindness you begin by feeling kind towards yourself, which some people find very difficult. If so, it's best to stay with practising a feeling of kindness towards yourself, until you begin to feel comfortable with it. Then you can expand it.

Here is a short meditation on kindness:

> Simply repeat, either out loud or silently to yourself, the following statements. (*These words are only a suggestion—you might find other words that you prefer.*)
> May I be filled with kindness.
> May I be well.
> May I be peaceful and at ease.
> May I be happy.
> (And then you can open this up to include everyone.)
> May everyone be filled with kindness.
> May everyone be well.
> May everyone be peaceful and at ease.
> May everyone be happy.

Compassion

The word *compassion* is derived from Latin and it means to be "with the passion". In this context, the meaning of the word *passion* is suffering. So it means the ability to accept pain as a fact of life—both in your own life and in the lives of others. This takes emotional strength and resources, and meditating on compassion is a conscious way to build in these resources.

All pain is a form of warning—it's the body's way to protect itself by warning that a limit has been, or is about to be, breached. This can happen psychologically, emotionally, and physically but the process is exactly the same. When we experience pain it invariably means we didn't see something, for example, the real needs of the body. We tend to override our feelings to push on and get things done, instead of working *with* our bodies. We expect them to just be there, like a machine, and perform to our expectations. However, the minor warnings of pain increase until we are brought to a standstill.

By meditating on compassion you can build in the strength and confidence to become aware of these signs of wear and tear. It's much easier to deal with in the early stages than when they are full-blown. Any car mechanic would take this for granted!

Compassion is understanding the limits that a human body and living in communities place on us and understanding that for life to exist, there must be differentiation, contrast and diversity. Knowing where the limits and boundaries are and respecting them provides the basis for being able to communicate skillfully.

Although this sounds very philosophic, we take it for granted every time we play sport, dance, or play music. The first thing we do is decide where the boundaries are going to be—it's impossible to play a game like football until this has been decided—then there are the rules of the game. These things define the limits. To have a game, all the participants have to agree to the rules and boundaries.

When we communicate, we use language and this too has its rules and boundaries. When these have been established and we respect each other's limits, the game can begin. We can dance together— communicate with and open to the feelings of others. This is the essence of compassion.

One way to meditate on compassion is to use the mantra **OM MANI PADME HUM**.

While saying the mantra imagine a large, while flower in your heart centre. Resting on this is a red jewel. From the jewel light radiates through your body—soft pink or the shimmering light of a rainbow.

If you wish, expand the light as far as you can imagine.

You can also use the word **LOVE** to meditate on compassion.

When I first began working with students and clients, teaching them how to meditate, the most important thing I could do initially was to listen—to open my mind and free it from all my ideas, so that I could actually *hear* what the other person was saying. This is not easy, because we are used to waiting until the other person stops talking to say what we want to say, so we are focusing on our own point of view. I found that doing the mantra of compassion was the best way to do let go of my point of view.

If I concentrated carefully on every word said, I missed the tone of voice, movements of the body and look in the eyes, so completely missed the emotion, expression and actual inner experience of the other person. I was still thinking, and so looking at the situation from my point of view.

Saying the mantra took me directly out of this bias, and completely opened my mind. It was a little unnerving at first because I thought I wouldn't have any idea how to respond without thinking. But I discovered that although I couldn't plan my response, a response would be there—almost of its own accord.

I then understood how communication is a form of compassion, because I could see the reaction of the student or client—their surprise and relief that somebody wasn't just serving up a point of view, but had opened to what they were actually experiencing. This was all that was needed because then they could hear and feel what they were saying rather than defending it against someone else.

Whenever I'm in an emotionally-charged situation, where people are angry, pained, frustrated or panicked, and the temptation to lose my cool is ever-present, repeating the mantra silently brings me to a calm, clear state. It takes me out of my mind, where thoughts are ready to pitch in and engage or attempt to solve it all, straight back to my body. Then they are connected, so the mind and body are able to work together. The jewel of the mind is resting in the open flower of the body.

Sharing joy

Loving someone is an extremely energising experience—it takes you out of yourself as you open up to the life experience, feelings and views of someone else. Sharing their happiness is joy and your heart has to be open to someone to share their joy. If it isn't, being with someone who is happy, either in themselves or about something that has happened in their lives, will make you jealous.

Joy is also experienced physically, because it is a form of relaxation as the tension in your body is released. For example, when you laugh, the muscles around your belly tense up, then let go and relax. This is why a good belly laugh is so healthy—one Zen teacher made it a key meditation! After you laugh, you breathe deeply into your belly, which opens your diaphragm and replaces the stale air at the bottom of your lungs.

Joy is the state of mind we experience when we contain energy in our bodies, allow it to build up and then release it. This process is outlined in the **Three C Technique**. By **Catching the moment**, you gather the energy together, then, by **Clearing the space** using meditation, you contain and concentrate the energy. This enables you to understand what you want to do and make a clear decision about how to use it. By **Changing the habit**, you can release the energy in a directed way instead of through habit.

As this energy releases it can be extremely creative—it can create completely new perspectives, create art and science, or build and regenerate relationships. Releasing energy through joy is the same as the release of a bud's energy as it opens and blossoms.

So joy is the creativity and sheer vitality we feel when joining in the dance of life; when sharing with someone we know and love, or meeting with someone who just happens to be passing through our lives. From this heart-space you can celebrate the diversity and abundance of life, the energy and exuberance, the thrill and ecstasy. Instead of restricting your life to a bland homogeneity you can, through meditating on joy, stretch your emotions and allow yourself to respond to the offer of being a partner in the dance with those around you.

> I believe my music teacher Olivier Messiaen encapsulated this feeling beautifully in the music and title of one of the movements of a major orchestral piece, *The Joy of the Blood of the Stars*. You can envisage the dance of joy on a universal stage and the play of energy on an enormous scale as stars and galaxies whirl through space, being created and destroyed. He thought joy was one of the most important things to express in music.

Meditating on joy also enables you to recognise joy in others and let go of the defences that prevent you from joining in. Recognising joy in others helps you to recognise and cultivate joy in yourself. In self-contained joy, you experience the bliss of your heart and mind opening, meeting and dancing. When sharing joy with others, the joy is an expression of meeting in that heart-space.

> A good way to enhance the practice of this meditation is to test whether you can maintain interest and pleasure in someone else's joy and success, or whether you begin to feel jealous of them. Jealousy is a particularly valuable emotion because you know immediately what you really want when you experience it.
>
> As soon as you feel jealous, the most skillful thing to do is completely accept it, then allow yourself to feel what the other person is feeling. Like all pain, jealousy is a warning: it means you are denying that feeling in yourself. You can train yourself to share in joy and vitality, and then you have the resources to give joy.

You can just repeat the word **JOY** to yourself.

More formally, you can use a mantra:

AHAM MAHA SUKHAM.

Pronounced: **AH-HUM MAR-HA SOOKHUM**

Rhythm: **Ah HUM Ma HA SookHUM**

This is the signature mantra for the Lifeflow Meditation Centre. It means, "I am great joy".

Balance and equanimity

In our culture we don't usually associate balance and equanimity with love. However, knowing how to find and maintain our balance is a fundamental requirement for understanding our inner life and developing emotional intelligence. Because every healthy mental and emotional state we experience is grounded in balance, it is also a key factor in our experience and expression of love.

The word *equanimity* literally means "equal mind", (from *aequus* "equal", and *animus* "mind"). Equanimity is the state of mind in which you can be equal with everything that comes your way; it's where your mind retains its balance and you can keep your cool. The ability to maintain this while experiencing powerful emotions like joy, sadness, deep affection, compassion, passion or sympathy is a true sign of love because one of the major symptoms of any loving emotion is a tendency to cling.

Because love feels so good, we want it to last—and at that moment we become stuck. Becoming emotionally attached to the point of dependence, and then clinging to the person or situation we love, is where all love is eventually destroyed. Clinging to someone or something prevents us from seeing them clearly—we become fixated on our idea of what they should be. The dance between us then grinds to a halt, because we are no longer moving in tune with them but are focused on our idea of what they should be. Anger can then take over as they do not conform to what we want, and this can eventually turn to hatred.

Equanimity is the wisdom aspect of love; it has no emotion associated with it because it is based on the mind being still. You can maintain a quality of clear awareness at the core of loving emotions and this quality of clarity makes them healthy. This is the only way to be free from the expectations we normally bring to our relationships, and freeing others from our expectations can be one of the kindest things we bring to them.

A good meditation to create balance is the simple three-syllable mantra, **OM AH HUM**. The syllable **OM** is focused in the head, **AH** is focused in the throat, and **HUM** is focused in the heart.

As you say this mantra, follow the sounds from your head to your heart while you say them silently or out loud.

If you like working with colour, say **OM** while visualising a white light in the forehead, **AH** while visualising a red light in the throat, and **HUM** while visualising a deep blue light in the middle of the chest—in the heart centre.

You can use the following meditation to contemplate the states of love—say the phrases out loud or silently to yourself.

May I be free from clinging and rejection and may I maintain myself happily.

May everyone have happiness and the causes of happiness.

May everyone be free from sorrow and the causes of sorrow.

May everyone share in the joy of life.

May everyone be free from clinging to those they love and indifference to others.

And know the precious quality of all life.

Food

Eating

Meditating on eating is a very direct way to keep in touch with the body and senses. Over the last few decades there has been a marked shift in emphasis from the taste, texture and seasonal and local variability of food to its visual appearance and year-round availability. This might explain why talking about and looking at food can take over from actually tasting it.

I remember revelling in the taste of fresh apricots straight off the tree as a child, with the juice running down my face. An entire generation of children has now grown up without this experience. Apricots from the supermarket bear no resemblance to what I remember. Neither do peaches, plums, nectarines or tomatoes. Instead of being ripe and juicy, they are hard and tasteless in spite of their visual appearance and the claims of freshness.

To meditate on food:

> Allow yourself to slow down and hold the food in your hand or on your fork, allowing its aroma to soak into your nostrils, and noticing its shape and colour. Then, when you place it in your mouth, hold it on your tongue for a while, feeling its texture and letting the taste spread through your whole mouth.
>
> Then chew the food and feel what it is like when you swallow. See if you can feel your whole body responding to what you have eaten.

Going to the toilet

The other side of meditating on food is going to the toilet. The original Buddhist monks, "wanderers", lived in the open and so defecating and urinating into the earth were a natural part of their meditative day.

Indigenous cultures, being much more in touch with their bodies and the earth, also accepted this as a natural part of their lives. Western culture, on the whole, doesn't, so enormous resources are poured into hiding it. An engineer told me that all of civil engineering was a process of connecting bums to the sea!

> Take time to observe your urine and faeces; they are a good indicator of the state of your health.
>
> Feel your body respond as you urinate and defecate—notice the relief and relaxation. Allow yourself to open to the feeling of letting go at this visceral level; it can become blissful to the point of ecstasy.
>
> Going to the toilet at work lends itself perfectly to a short moment of relaxation and the chance to balance yourself. You can experience the pleasure of letting go.

Elements of the body

Analysing the elements of your body is a very active form of meditation because it deliberately uses your thinking. The aim of this is to see your body as a constantly changing process rather than a fixed, solid entity. You may wish to read the basic ideas of physics and chemistry—just to have some working knowledge of the processes and elements that make up our bodies.

Analysing your own body helps you to see where it came from, where it is now and where it is going. You see how totally dependent your body is on the network that supports it—its life, the lives of others and the environment around you are completely interdependent.

To meditate on your body:

> While seated, hold your hands in your lap, one underneath the other, palms facing up so you can focus comfortably on the palm of one hand.
>
> Allow everything you notice and all the associations you have to fill your mind. Notice the shape, lines, skin colour and texture.
>
> Then let your mind go back in time so you have a feeling for your hand when it was young. Now imagine it in the womb and still a part of your mother's body.
>
> Keep going back into how it evolved and how it formed from the elements of the earth.
>
> Then move to its future—see it growing older and eventually dying and returning to those elements from which it was made.

You can also focus on the detail when you are meditating on a visual object such as a piece of fruit, leaf, feather, or a rock.

> Instead of letting your eyes rest gently on the object, focus on each detail, bringing them to mind, deliberately analysing all the elements of the object.
>
> You can see the common elements between your own body and the visual object; how they survive within the same limits and operate under the same laws.

You can begin to see your body as part of the universe and the universe in your body. For example, you can see the leaf of a tree and your body as part of the earth and so the leaf in your body and your body in the leaf. You can get a feeling for this vast process we call life.

The infinite absorptions

The infinite states of absorption are the four meditation objects that have no form, so they are often called the *formless states*. They are detailed in Chapter 12 so only briefly summarised here.

The infinite absorptions are universal intuitive experiences that explore the limits of human consciousness. As you rest in the fourth level of absorption your mind becomes so balanced and your concentration so fine that you can experience these subtle states. The infinite absorptions arise in a particular order and begin with the experience of **infinite space**.

Infinite space

This is a very refined and subtle meditation and I only recommend it if you have been practising for at least a year and have a teacher to guide you.

> Use your favourite meditation to bring yourself to an absorbed state.
>
> Then visualise a column of light through the centre of your body and follow your breathing into the heart or navel centre to help you establish the second and then the third levels of absorption.
>
> To sustain the third level, slightly slow down the in-breath and focus it into the heart or navel centre. As you breathe out, allow the body boundaries to dissolve, and a feeling of heaviness and sinking to permeate your body.
>
> To establish the fourth level, breathe into the navel centre and then shift your focus to the out-breath, following each breath to the end of the breath.
>
> Let the out-breath slow down, so you can rest in the pause at the end of the out-breath.
>
> When you notice your breathing has become so fine and shallow that you hardly breathe in, your breath will pause. You can feel the steady, balanced state of this level of absorption—it is extremely still and solid.
>
> To experience infinite space, let go of focusing on your breath and allow your mind to open and expand. You can either feel the space around you and let your mind rest in space, or meditate on the idea of space. You allow the form of breathing and the boundaries of your mind to dissolve, so you can literally feel your mind expanding into space.

Infinite consciousness, sphere of nothingness, the boundary of perception

The remaining formless states are consecutive and arise naturally once your mind has reached the level of **infinite space**. Normally you would need to be in retreat for this to happen. Refer back to Chapter 12 for descriptions of these states.

Matching meditation with personality type and level of concentration or absorption

Use the following chart to match each meditation object with the personality types discussed in Chapter 21, and to see how far each meditation object will take you. Refer back to Chapter 5 for the deepening stages of meditation, or Chapter 12 for the levels of absorption.

Meditation object	Best for personality type	Level of concentration or absorption
The four elements: earth, water, fire, wind	All personality types	Fourth level of absorption
Colours	Stepping back	Fourth level of absorption
Space	All personality types	Fourth level of absorption
Light and consciousness	All personality types	Fourth level of absorption
Meditating on death directly	Moving forward	First level of absorption
Contemplating death	All personality types	First deepening stage of meditation
Contemplating the body	Moving forward	First level of absorption
Contemplating openness	All personality types	First deepening stage of meditation
Contemplating peace	All personality types	First deepening stage of meditation
Contemplating the foundation of the mind	All personality types	First deepening stage of meditation
Visualisations	All personality types but especially moving forward	First or second level of absorption
Breathing	All personality types but especially staying still	Fourth level of absorption and can then open up awareness or insight, or lead you into the infinite absorptions
Four states of love	Stepping back	Kindness, compassion and joy will take you to the third level of absorption, and equanimity to the fourth level of absorption.
Physical sensations of eating	Stepping back	First level of absorption
Physical sensations of going to the toilet	Moving forward	First level of absorption
Analysing elements of the body	Moving forward	First deepening stage of meditation and perhaps the first level of absorption
Meditating on the body	All personality types	First level of absorption
Infinite absorptions	All personality types	The infinite absorptions are a development of the fourth level of absorption.

The next chapter explores the different paths of meditation, which are based on how people process information.

Chapter 23: The different paths of meditation

If we try to learn something without being aware of our natural talents and abilities, we waste time and energy attempting to learn in ways that don't suit us.

Chapter 21 described personality types which were classified according to the natural reaction people have to an object. The meditation tradition also recognised that people come to understand things in their own way, depending on their natural abilities. Knowing that we all learn differently can be a revelation and a great relief to many people.

This chapter describes three different meditation paths and personality types based on how people *process information*—how they understand the world. Like the typology based on how people respond to an object, this has been part of the tradition for thousands of years. It's a very effective way to understand how different people view the world and communicate—so effective that it was rediscovered last century by Jung and in Neuro-Linguistic Programming (NLP).

The do-er, the feeler, the thinker

The three meditation paths are learning through senses, learning through feelings and learning through thinking. I call them **the do-er—the sensing type, the lover—the feeling type** and **the seer—the intuitive-thinking type.**

As with all learning skills, if you try to learn something without being aware of your natural abilities and skills, you waste an enormous amount of time and energy attempting to learn in ways that don't suit you.

The do-er—the sensing type

The first personality type identifies with their bodies and is very aware of their senses. They are people of action who learn through doing, so they are "hands on" people and nothing will make sense to them until they have got the feel of it and tried it out to see what it does. They don't like to dwell on abstract concepts—this is alien territory for them.

What is *physical* is what is real for them. In tantric terms they are gut people because the focus of the physical body is the navel centre. So they usually have plenty of guts, will pitch in physically and have a go. They see with their bodies and it's only through the physical reaction of their bodies that they "get it".

The path of body-witness

The path of the do-er is called the path of "body-witness". All their experiences in meditation will be played out physically. The knots, tensions, pains and conflicts that are part of everyone's life will manifest in their bodies. This can be very unnerving if they are not guided by someone who understands what is happening. They will be convinced that things are going very wrong; that they have contracted all kinds of illnesses so rush to the doctor.

> I've had many people referred who have done the rounds of doctors, psychologists and psychiatrists, gaining no understanding or satisfaction. They really are experiencing these things; but the health professionals are also right: there is nothing really wrong with them from a medical point of view. However, from the point of view of meditation, it was obvious what was happening. The source of their experiences was the *energy body*. When they tried exercises that allowed them to open up to their inner experience, they could see clearly what their bodies were attempting to tell them. The physical symptoms then disappeared.
>
> If anyone comes to me with these kinds of symptoms I always suggest, if they have not already done so, that they check everything with a doctor. If they come up with a clean bill of health, it is clear where the problem lies.

The ecstasies are also played out in the body—their bodies will shake and tremble as knots of tension undo. The joy and rapture of meditation will be a direct physical experience for them as it vibrates through their bodies.

This can also be referred to as "the wet path" because it uses up tissues and toilet paper as orifices at both ends completely let go. Releasing knots, tension and pain through tears, vomiting and diarrhea is the only way the body knows how—and it leaves a feeling of complete relief.

The path of form

In meditation practice the do-er will focus on yoga—both physical yoga and tantra (energy body yoga), and also movement meditation because these provide plenty to do. They can stretch their bodies to the limit, and learn how to stretch the inner body—the energy body.

This path is also called "the path of form" because you work with objects that have a shape: your physical body and energy body. Do-ers need to learn how to focus their energies, open chakras and explore them, work with the channels, winds and currents of their energy body, and develop the power to build and shape both bodies. They need to be kept busy, feel productive, and see results.

The realisation of the do-er

When this path comes to fruition, do-ers see that pain and conflict, agony and ecstasy, no matter how long they last or how dramatic, are not personal. They are just part of the package when you have a body. Every form of life struggles to survive and suffers conflict—the do-er experiences this in their own body.

Just as they are prepared to work their bodies hard to achieve a goal, they see that the pain of stretching themselves emotionally is the same. They see that their emotional pain has nothing to do with being bad, or that anything has gone wrong, it's just work, like any kind of work. They don't feel the need to control everything any more. From this comes the moment of direct insight where they see and experience the universal law in which all their experience rests.

Do-ers reach this insight by developing powers of calm and concentration to the point where they can sustain the states of absorption and enter the infinite absorptions. This comes through working with their bodies, outer and inner, until they can maintain their physical balance and be still, focused and concentrated. It's a path where they sweat to stay still—no pain, no gain. They feel the satisfaction of hard work, so the rewards and achievements are also deeply satisfying. They have developed real inner power.

The lover—the feeling type

This personality type identifies with their emotions; reality is their feelings and they experience this through relationship. They feel everything deeply, are passionate about things, fall in love constantly and are devoted. Their life is dominated by how they feel about themselves and other people, and how other people feel about them. They love communicating, and are usually very skilled at it, either through inner work like art or literature, or by being good listeners and talkers. The feeling type also inspires devotion—they can be charismatic so they make excellent teachers, performers and politicians.

> A famous Australian talk-back host, whose program ran for thirty years once said that if he was forced to stop he would die. It didn't matter whether he was nice or rude and insulting, listeners couldn't get enough. I once heard someone ring in to complain (because he called one of the callers stupid), who said that if *he* were called stupid he would sue. The radio star immediately said, "You're stupid—now sue me!" Amazingly they continued to chat for five minutes without any hard feelings. Listeners felt their existence had been confirmed; that they had been touched and communicated with.

The aim of this type is to "feel at one with", "feel connected to" or "be in union with" others, the world and perhaps the universe. They have no sense of logic and do not necessarily take any notice of facts, because they follow their feelings. If they are spiritually inclined, the idea of God has meaning, because for them it is something they can feel.

In tantric terms they are heart people, because the heart is the centre of our emotional and feeling life. They look for someone or something they can be devoted to and surrender to, so they can experience being absorbed in something bigger than themselves. They can empathise strongly with others and lose themselves completely in devotion to an art, cause or helping others. Their discipline is one of committing themselves to someone or something, and taking on the work of the inner life.

The path of the devotee
In meditation, the path of the feeling type is called "the path of the devotee". As someone follows this path they develop the kind of emotional strength that reveals itself as genuine confidence. They develop complete trust.

Although all three meditation paths encompass the process of moving beyond your identity and allowing yourself to be absorbed by something bigger than yourself, for the devotee this needs to be a relationship they can *feel*. So they are particularly drawn to religious devotion or guru devotion. It's a shame there has been such a history of abuse around this, because it is a necessary process for the devoted type.

In the training of classical music there is a long tradition of students being completely devoted to their teachers. A student-teacher relationship based on devotion needs a real body of work to sustain it, and this is why in music it can be so productive and healthy. The same thing can happen between a student and sports coach or in a relationship with a mentor.

The path of devotion goes wrong when there is no work, and the devotee believes all they have to do is feel devoted. This is a form of emotional laziness and any minister, priest, guru or teacher who encourages this betrays not only the faithful, the devotee or the student, but also the path of devotion.

The classical meditation tradition assumed that everyone involved had taken up the practice of meditation so was training their mind and emotions. There was a body of work to be completed, and the teacher checked this work and assisted the student to attain their own experiences and realisations—all of which could be tested. Devotion needed to be balanced by reason and inquiry, so there was never any question of blind faith.

Naturally this still holds. A meditation teacher needs to make it clear that without a regular practice and commitment to sustaining a body of work, it is not possible to train the mind. It is the same for any true discipline and this is what keeps a discipline alive and healthy. There is then a real dialogue between teacher and student, because each student will bring their own experience, questions and understanding to the work, adding to it and helping to shape it, as in the arts and sciences. The work and training are not fixed and limited for all time, but are a living, constantly growing organism that is renewed, tested and shaped by each generation.

This type is prepared to stretch the envelope emotionally and go where others fear to tread. For example, they can be intimate, loving and tender one moment, and create extreme emotional and hysterical scenes the next. Anyone who has worked in theatre or music understands this well. They will also experiment with their emotions by diving into "inappropriate" relationships and taking drugs.

They love a good emotional workout, and life is boring and dull unless this is happening. This is the path of "The Agony and the

Ecstasy". They will be ravished by love, as was Saint Theresa of Avila. They will weep tears of joy. If they do not learn some kind of emotional discipline, this type can go right off the deep end and become manic depressive—swinging from one emotional extreme to the other without any control. They are prone to dramatic gestures, and can swing to the point of suicide.

The path of form

In their meditation practice, the lover will initially tend to focus on visualisation and mantra, because here you work with relationship. These techniques build a relationship with all the different states of mind and emotions we experience. Lovers explore all the different ways it is possible to relate to others, so develop finely honed skills of communication.

Communication is the foundation of compassion, so the feeling type is usually very attracted to meditations concentrating on developing compassion, kindness and love. In following "the path of form", the feeling type will also work with Tantra, which brings together the bliss in the body and spacious openness in the mind.

The realisation of the lover

As a person who identifies with their feelings tends to see them as solid and lasting, their conflicts are played out in their emotions. Just as the do-er experiences reality in their bodies and doesn't become aware of their own pain or a painful situation until it becomes physical, a lover only becomes aware of conflict and pain when they feel it in their emotions.

However, by learning to sit still with their emotions and with guidance from a teacher to whom they are devoted, they begin to see past their seeming permanence. Working with the emotional variations of visualisation and mantra, they expand the variety of their emotional experience, and come to see the shifts and changes in emotions. Working with a teacher as the partner in their emotional exploration, they realise that the teacher doesn't seem to be thrown around by emotions, as they would expect. They become able to remain balanced and calm in the face of emotional storms.

This brings them to see directly, and experience emotionally, the fact that every emotion, no matter how powerful, subsides of its own accord. It will always end by balancing itself and resting in the space and openness of a balanced mind. Lovers come to see that this is a universal law that applies to everything and the solid core of confidence they can develop rests on directly experiencing this. They are freed from emotional conflict through developing confidence.

The seer—the intuitive-thinking type

This personality type identifies with their thinking. This is not the kind of thinking that leads to organisational skills or business management, but to asking the big questions—where things come from and where they go, how and why we happen to be here, who we are, how the mind and universe work. They have a natural curiosity about the processes of the mind itself. The seer is the visionary; someone who can grasp the big picture and see causes and consequences well into the past and future.

Consciousness also interests them intensely and to the seer this concept is very real. They seek to be conscious and to understand consciousness. Abstract concepts are their territory and they revel in them—the bigger the better. Because they identify with clear thinking, they are the eggheads of society, so in tantric terms they are focused in the head centre.

The path of wisdom

In the tradition this path is called "the path of wisdom", the path of seeing. The seer aims to be the sage—the one who knows. Seers identify with what they know; they are not necessarily likeable, and don't seek to be liked—it's not important to them. Of paramount importance is that things are clear and they understand them.

They tend not to be interested in their bodies and are certainly not swayed by their emotions. Things don't really register unless they are expressed in abstract terms, in concepts that can be discussed coolly and reasonably. Conflict and pain are experienced in their minds as they do battle with the contradictions inherent in our thought processes.

They drive lovers completely mad because they are so "cold" and do-ers find them dry, boring and out of touch with real life. Meanwhile, seers can't understand why lovers and do-ers don't see clearly when things have been explained so reasonably.

This is also called "the dry path" (as distinct from "the wet path" of the do-er) because it is dry and cool—detached from the world, looking at it dispassionately and working out why things are they way they are, just like the Buddha, or a physics professor.

If your main preoccupation is tracking cause and effect to understand the laws of the universe or the cause of human suffering, you can't do it if you don't remain cool and self-contained. You simply don't have the energy to develop the degree of concentration required. And discovering these laws has been of enormous benefit to humankind. Compassion is not necessarily warm, it can be cool, and the compassion of the seer is a cool compassion.

The path of non-form

Unlike do-ers and lovers, the intuitive-thinking type doesn't work through the path of form at all. Although they can develop the absorptions, they don't need to because they have the mental stability to work things out in their heads.

> A friend who gained his Masters in mathematics from Cambridge University told me he found doing mathematical problems on paper far too slow because, having developed the skill of meditation over a number of years, he found it much easier to visualise the problem in his head, work out the solution, and write it down afterwards!

The seer works through the "path of non-form". They don't stretch their muscles or emotions, but they stretch their mind. They work by following the mind wherever it goes—so it's a path of awareness rather than a path of creation. The seer isn't interested in making things happen; they simply want to become aware of what is happening. Their path is one of awareness and mindfulness, and insight meditation is pretty well all they need. They are perfectly happy with the coolness and bareness of it.

The realisation of the seer

In the path of form you make effort physically and emotionally. The path of non-form is effortless in that you are just watching whatever happens in the mind until you go beyond all forms, stories and concepts and discover its innate space.

The seer is seeking ultimate truth. In the tradition there is a clear distinction made between *relative truth* and *ultimate truth*. *Relative truth* deals with the reality of the world as we know it—everything that exists can only exist under certain conditions, in relation to everything else. Science has thoroughly explored this world of relativity. *Ultimate truth* deals with the fundamental facts of existence.

Seers' minds open up to the realisation of fundamental awareness, of openness and emptiness. They discover ultimate truth by following their minds and thought processes, until they discover the ledge—the limit of thought. They discover that knowledge is really a process of understanding where the limits are, of *knowing the **ledges***. They are freed from the conflict inherent in the process of thinking (working with concepts that inevitably contradict each other) by seeing directly through the process of thinking itself.

They discover that not only is thought innately empty of any building block, but so is everything else; nothing has a solid core or base, and the foundation of everything is openness or space.

The mixture

As we are all a bit of a mixture when it comes to personality types, a balanced path will tend to incorporate elements of all three paths, which is what we teach at Lifeflow. Every student quickly finds where their natural abilities lie and follows the path which suits them. However, seers need some physical and emotional stretching to keep their bodies and hearts in shape. Do-ers and lovers both need to learn how to think clearly, and lovers find that physical exercise keeps their emotional excesses in check.

So each personality type can tailor a path to suit their individual needs. For example, I am definitely not physically inclined but have found that physical exercises, swimming, walking and bike riding have been of enormous value. I could never take yoga to the level of a do-er, but I enjoy some of the basic stretches and they keep me in good health.

> After working as a concert pianist, I was definitely following the path of the lover. However, when I began meditating my teacher said that I had "done mantra". I gradually discovered that he meant I had completed the path of form appropriate to my type. He then took me straight into the dry path—to insight. I discovered the importance of the different paths through teaching people who couldn't seem to do what came naturally to me.

Everyone needs to work initially with some of the path of form and everyone will eventually enter the path of non-form. Almost all of the great teachers and practitioners in the lineage practised both—

including the Buddha. It's a matter of how the balance is struck and where the talents and abilities lie. The paths converge when someone has attained a certain level of work and understanding.

The three bodies

As discussed earlier, in Tantra there are three bodies to work with: the **physical body**, the **mental body** and the **energy body**. Let's examine this structure in more detail.

The physical body

When we refer to our body, we are discussing our *physical body*. Our culture has studied it thoroughly, and developed a tradition of medicine and science which encompasses the entire range of physical knowledge from healing broken limbs to microbiology and neuroscience.

However, Tantra defines a body as anything that has a shape or form and a beginning and an end. If you look around at the objects in your room: this book you are reading, the chairs and tables, lights, glasses and everything else, they all have a shape, a beginning and an end. Because they have a form, they exist in time and space, and having been created, will eventually disintegrate. So the definition holds for physical objects. Let's look at our thoughts.

The mental body

If you examine any thought you will discover that you experience it as an image or a word. An image definitely has a shape, and so a beginning and an end—as does a word. So the definition holds for thoughts. Tantra considers our whole range of mental processes— thoughts, images, conversations and memories—as a body. In the West, we use this concept when we speak of a *body of knowledge*. In Tantra this is called the *mental body*.

We are all familiar with our mental processes and thoughts and are well trained to look after our physical bodies. However, there is one more body.

The energy body

Tantra calls this last body the *energy body*. It consists of all the inner sensations and emotions we experience. If you watch any sensation or emotion you will find it has a specific location in your physical body. It also has a beginning and an end and, when you examine it closely, a form. This surprises people until they are asked to draw or paint an emotion, and find they can.

In the West, it is only recently that the energy body has been taken seriously—it was previously dismissed as imagination or vague emotions—and studied in natural medicine, where it is sometimes called the *energetic body*. The Tantric tradition accepts all three bodies and has made a specialised study of the energy body.

We discuss our energies all the time without noticing what we are saying. For example, we are *full of energy*, or *lacking in energy*. We have *butterflies in the stomach, broken hearts, choked up throats* and headaches of all kinds. The Tantric tradition understands what causes these things, how they work and how to heal them.

Maintaining physical, emotional and mental health

The concept of the three bodies allows us to view our mental and emotional lives quite differently. For example, we take for granted that our physical bodies need to be fed, so we have a number of meals each day. However, all of our aspects—physical, emotional and mental—follow the same laws. As they are all bodies, they all need to be fed to remain healthy. At some level we know this because we talk about *food for the soul* and *food for the mind*.

At school we learn how to read and write and fill our minds with knowledge, learning ideas and concepts. Our thinking could not operate without ideas and concepts—these are what feed our mental bodies and thoughts.

If you meet someone who is starved of ideas and doesn't know how to feed themselves on this level you will see all the symptoms of hunger. For example, an elderly person who has depended on local or family gossip to feed their minds but is now isolated in a nursing home, will languish for want of mental nourishment. When someone visits them they are hungry for the latest gossip.

In Tantra it is understood that the energy body is fed by the breath. This is a very new idea for us and you might think "Well, we all breathe". However, we have to know how to work with the breath and how to prepare it, in the same way that we prepare food for our physical bodies.

Many people who work with the heart—therapists, counsellors, doctors etc.—become emotionally drained, literally drained of energy, because they have no idea how to feed their energy body. When people learn how to feed themselves with their breath it is a revelation as their energies recover.

Three bodies and three types

Each personality type will tend to focus their attention, work and identities on one of these three bodies. This shapes their view of themselves, the world and what is real for them. Do-ers will become very aware of their physical health and nourishment. Their physical body will be the focus of their meditation. Lovers will seek to feed themselves spiritually so will maintain their energy body through meditation, incorporating breathing exercises into their practice. And seers will look to the ideas and concepts in the teaching to feed their mental body.

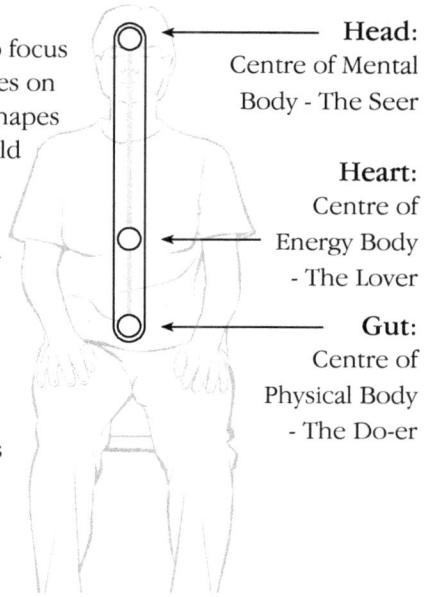

Head:
Centre of Mental
Body - The Seer

Heart:
Centre of
Energy Body
- The Lover

Gut:
Centre of
Physical Body
- The Do-er

The three types rediscovered in Neuro-Linguistic Programming

In the 20th century, as the discipline of psychology gradually developed, the idea of personality types came to be taken more seriously. Jung's work was adapted to create the Myer-Briggs test, which could reveal a person's type reasonably accurately. It is used extensively in business, recruitment and psychology.

Although they were not psychologists, two academics, Bandler and Grinder, searched for a way to achieve excellence efficiently and created a system called Neuro-Linguistic Programming (NLP)[21]. They discovered that people process information in three ways—visually, aurally or kinaesthetically (through the sensations in their bodies). Therefore, people speak one of three kinds of languages, and for effective communication, it is essential to know which language a person is using.

They rediscovered the same typing system that has been an integral part of the meditation tradition for thousands of years, by using the same technique—close observation and testing their hypotheses by gradually removing the variables.

The person who processes information visually is the intuitive-thinking type. These people work mainly through images in their heads. They tend to speak quickly to keep up with the flow of images, and their voices are consequently pitched in their heads and rather dry.

Note that I called this type the seer and visionary—these are visual words, which are part of the language of this type. The visual type "Sees what you mean", "Looks closely at things", "Sees eye to eye", and can "Shed light on things".

The aural type is the same as the feeling type—the lover—of the meditation tradition. These people process information through sound and work through words, so their path is mantra and visualisation, because they need to have a conversation with someone. They "Hear what you mean", "Live in harmony", "Hear something loud and clear" and for them something can "Ring a bell".

They listen to their own inner conversation, to others and to their bodies. As NLP points out, their voices resonate in their chest—they are more embodied than the visual type. Their voices are generally warm and inviting.

The kinaesthetic type is the same as the sensing type of meditation––the do-er. These people process information through the sensations they experience in their bodies so their path includes the yogas of tantra and movement meditation. Their language reflects this; they "Get in touch with you", "Feel something in their bones", ask you to "Hold on a second" and will notice that something just "Scratches the surface". Their voices resonate in their belly and can, if needed, really pack a punch.

The next chapter revisits the four streams of meditation (briefly outlined in the introduction), and explores how they work together and are integrated with everyday life.

Chapter 24: The four streams of meditation

You develop Calm and Concentration and Insight by sitting still. The streams of Tantra and Ethics are the direct application of meditation.

In the introduction to this book I briefly outlined the four streams of the meditation tradition: Calm and Concentration, Insight, Ethics and Tantra. This chapter discusses each stream in detail and explains how they work together.

Calm and Concentration

The first meditation stream is **Calm and Concentration**. Most meditation exercises are aimed at developing and sustaining a state where the mind, emotions and body are completely balanced and connected. This is essential for all meditation practice—nothing can be achieved without this state of balance.

As we have seen, the absorptions can be developed from a light state of absorption where you are still thinking, through to a state where your whole mind and body are so balanced that even your breathing pauses. On this basis your mind can open up to experiences of consciousness beyond our normal limits of perception, or it can open up to insight.

Insight

While meditations for developing calm and concentration use a meditation object to allow the mind to rest and become still, **Insight** meditation is a process of following your mind wherever its focus goes—to whatever object is in the mind. Keeping your mind focused on whatever is happening, so that your focus is constantly moving from object to object is called *mindfulness*.

The Insight stream trains both mindfulness and awareness. Deep stages of absorption become counterproductive because they are so still and inner-oriented. For Insight meditation only a light state of absorption is needed, because it is aimed at using our thinking effectively and keeping it linked to what we are actually experiencing with our senses. So it's designed to keep our minds and bodies connected.

Seeing things as they are

The ultimate aim of Insight meditation is to see everything as it actually is, as distinct from what we think, hope or fear might be happening. This means keeping what we are experiencing and seeing *free from our own expectations*, which is not as easy as it might sound.

We usually assume that we do see things as they are. How else could we see them? Well, apart from the fact that our senses operate within a limited range of experience, there is the added limitation that we see everything according to how we have been taught to name it. Our perceptions are shaped by our language, culture, parents, schooling and so on.

For example, I love classical music and find it a rich expression of our inner emotions, but I know people who hate classical music—they find it unutterably boring. As far as they are concerned, nothing is happening over an awfully long period of time. I enjoy swimming and body surfing, but I have friends who are serious surfers, and instead of finding huge surf exhilarating as they do, I find it daunting and exhausting.

These are straightforward examples of how our own conditioning and experience shape the way we see things. Insight meditation is designed to penetrate the veil of conditioning through which we see the world. We tend to see our conditioning as solid, reasonably stable and completely separate from ourselves, and never think to question these assumptions.

From the experience of direct seeing without any conditioned view––*seeing without naming*—the whole structure of Buddhist philosophy and psychology is built.

Watching without doing

The essence of Insight meditation is learning to just watch without needing to do anything, name what we are watching, or tell a story about it. We often find this very difficult, particularly when it comes to our own emotions and sensations, because we expect to control them. We can even feel a bit lazy because we're not doing anything about them. However, it's worth asking how we know what we are seeing if we never take the time to observe.

The foundation of Insight meditation is a calm and balanced state, so that we don't get emotionally caught, and can just watch. A typical exercise is just watching our everyday activities. For example:

Watch the action from beginning to end while drinking a cup of coffee.

Watch when you pick up the cup, when you move it to your lips, when you drink, and when you put the cup back on the table.

Keep your mind with the physical action throughout the whole movement.

The mind is full of the action

Keeping the mind with an action in this way is called *mindfulness*, because the mind has been focused on the action from beginning to end, so the *mind* has been *full* of the action. No other thoughts, conversations or side issues were present in the mind at that time.

Each time you do this exercise you will notice that the movements of your body are smooth, leaving you feeling very calm and satisfied. Your mind and body are connected for the whole of the action, so you feel the cup, its texture and temperature, really smell and taste the coffee, and your mind registers your body's sensations while drinking it.

Many disciplines like sport, music, art, science and the martial arts develop this quality of mindfulness, but it's amazing *how little we actually do this in our everyday lives*.

Awareness

Insight meditation is also designed to develop awareness. As with all meditation practices, we begin by focusing the mind on an object and holding it there so the mind and body become balanced and still. Mindfulness then keeps the focus right on the object so that the mind becomes full of the object, no matter where it goes—this is *one-pointed concentration*, the spotlight quality of the mind.

Awareness is developed by letting the mind open from this point. An exercise designed for this is to move the focus of the mind from the actual object to the space between you and the object, to meditate on space itself. This opens the mind to its floodlight quality, and it can be developed to a very high degree of concentration. It is *open* or *receptive concentration*.

The direct experience of the nature of the mind will arise from this form of concentration, and this is called Insight. Because it is based on open concentration, the instructions for Insight are to make no effort, let things come and go of their own accord, to allow the mind to rest in its natural state, and so on.

These instructions assume that you have achieved a high level of one-pointed concentration, and that your mind and body can be sustained in a balanced state. Then you give up focusing the mind on anything in particular—allowing it to rest in its balanced state. You maintain the state of just watching everything as it comes and goes. This brings the mind to a state of completely open awareness where nothing is more or less important than anything else. So you are developing the ability to *focus on nothing in particular* and be aware *of everything in general*.

Why do Insight meditation?
There is a very good reason for developing insight into the nature of our minds and seeing how our consciousness works. Many of the assumptions we have about our minds lead to quite a distorted view of reality. We assume that our minds are filled with thoughts, which are always there, and that we are a central figure in our minds, fixed and stable, totally separate from everything else in our minds.

This view creates exactly the same distortions in our inner reality as the earth-centred view did of our solar system. Insight into the nature of the mind is the direct experience of the open, clear, luminous state of awareness, which is the foundation of our minds. This can be compared with the space in which our planet, solar system and universe exist. We touch on this every time we meditate and bring our minds and bodies to a balanced state. *Insight is the direct seeing and experience of this space, this quality of awareness, along with the understanding of what it means.*

Tantra

The word *tantra* usually conjures up ideas about sex—tantric sex has become a fashion and many advertisements and books promote its benefits. This idea is not completely untrue but is a rather shallow reflection of one of the richest traditions in the East.

Naturally, a Tantric sex weekend would have its benefits. For those of us who have built-in guilt around sex (which includes most people raised in a Western culture), and for people who have tried everything and are looking to regenerate their sexual relationship, it would definitely get things moving along. However, this isn't what the stream of **Tantra** is for.

In Tantra, emotions and sensations are called the currents and winds of the body, and they are studied in the same way you would study the currents of the sea and winds of the atmosphere. Like yoga, which is designed to keep the body balanced and supple, Tantra provides techniques and exercises to keep our energies supple, balanced and alive. It taps directly into the life energy of the body and trains it. This is why it is associated with sex, because sexuality is one of the few experiences where people are directly in touch with their life energies, and experience the bliss and ecstasy they generate.

Tantra is designed to keep the mind and body integrated, from the root of our instincts to the warmth of our hearts and clarity of our minds. Tantric exercises are designed to consciously tap the driving force of our life energies, to strengthen the internal systems of the body to hold this amount of energy, and to use it to generate and sustain a state of bliss, ecstasy and clarity.

Bliss is the natural state of the body

Because Tantra is based on the development of Calm and Concentration and the realisation that everything is ephemeral and transparent, it works with the understanding that happiness is actually a state of mind. Tantric exercises therefore focus on working with emotions and states of mind. They provide a way to keep the mind and body fresh, alive, balanced and integrated no matter what the conditions and circumstances of life actually are.

Bliss is the natural state of the body, and the tragedy of human life is that to develop the skill of thinking, we have repressed this state, so most people don't feel anything most of the time. So they try to create bliss through buying something or going out, believing that they need to get something from outside and own it or eat it.

Tantra is a tool for drinking from the wellspring of our own lives. The word *tantra* means "thread" or "weaving", so Tantra is a tool for weaving together the threads of our lives, both internally and externally. It brings together all the disparate elements of our lives so that secular and sacred, instead of being separate and in conflict, are unified in a continuum of bliss and awareness.

No distinction between spiritual and material

So Tantra makes no distinction between spiritual and material. In this meditation stream, yearning, desire, lust, aggression, anger, jealousy and pride—all the powerful emotions that drive human life—are tapped and transformed. The poison is drunk, and the carefully constructed rules of what is and what isn't meditation are deconstructed.

The groin, heart and head are united, because they form one body and one mind. Heaven, earth and hell are united, because they are all products of our own states of mind. All the tantric exercises point to the fact that every emotion we experience, no matter how sublime or gross, is a different aspect of our life energy. In fact, every experience we have in the body (emotions, sensations, thoughts) is an interpretation of the way that energy is moving through the body. Fundamentally *it's all the same energy*.

The first steps in Tantra are learning to contain these forces and then balance and consciously direct them. Usually when we feel a strong emotion we can either repress or express it—either way the energy is lost and the intensity is frightening. The goal of Tantra is to be fearless in the face of the powerful forces that drive our lives, from the raw natural instincts to the refined, intense concentration of the mind.

Ethics—meditation in action

The final meditation stream is **Ethics**, which is concerned with applying the knowledge and experience derived from meditation to how we act. This stream focuses on how we move our bodies through the world and how we relate to others and the world around us.

Applying the knowledge and techniques of meditation to action has nothing to do with what we normally think of as ethics. It is the physical application of meditation, what we actually do in the thick of life experiences. It is not an intellectual or moralistic exercise, but a very practical one.

The basis of this stream is the ability to maintain balance, emotionally and mentally, even under the most demanding circumstances. The key to understanding this is the original meaning of the word usually translated as *ethics* in Buddhism. The word *Sila* means "coolness" and this is the aim of applying meditation to action—remaining "cool", no matter how mind-boiling the situation might be.

Understanding values—what they are and how they affect our actions—is a necessary part of the stream of Ethics.

How values affect decisions

Actions begin with decisions, and we are usually unaware that our values affect the decisions we make. In fact, our values are so ingrained, we are usually not aware of them at all. For example, they can range from believing that life is a matter of "dog eat dog", to believing that everyone is essentially good and it is only circumstances that cause some people to act without regard for others.

Our values represent our relationship with our bodies; they are an expression of our feelings, and feelings are the direct experience we have of our bodies. This is why it is necessary to become aware of our values when we apply meditation to what we actually do, because it's only with our bodies that we can do anything. Our feelings about ourselves and our lives shape the way we see the world and therefore the judgments at the base of our decisions and actions. Through meditation we can become aware of this process so both our feelings and the actual experience of our bodies can be integrated with our minds when we act.

Some people believe it is possible to be "value-free", but even the idea of something being value-free is a value. Every time we make any kind of decision we are judging that we prefer this over that, or we will go this way instead of that. So every decision, every judgment we make *is an expression of our inherent values.*

For example, where and how we live expresses our values. The West primarily values individuality, the East community. Science values truth, testing and repeatability. Business values profit—there is no confusion over this at all.

The stream of Ethics examines how we can use meditation to make decisions, by becoming aware of what our values actually are and testing them in everyday life, and by keeping our mental and emotional balance wherever we are.

> The success of a company I once worked with derived in large part from consciously adopting a set of values at incorporation. A friend of mine once said that greed, pure and simple, drives business, and this has a lot of truth in it. However, this company has developed a culture where there is genuine concern for the wellbeing of its employees, and this has resulted in a sense of participation, of concern for the company, and a strong sense of camaraderie, which have all played a large part in the company's success.

Moving from a state of balance

The aim of integrating meditation with our daily lives is to ensure that we develop the ability to move from a state of emotional and mental balance. By establishing balance before we act, we ensure that our minds, emotions and bodies are united and aimed in the same direction rather than the mind thinking about something else, the body running on ingrained habits, and the emotions registering the split between them.

This is integrated action; keeping mind and body together when making decisions and moving through everyday activities. It is also the art of acting mindfully, with the mind fully focused on what is being done. This undivided state is a state of integrity and this state of wholeness is the essential point of ethics. I like to describe it as *moving your body skillfully through the world*.

Bringing the four streams together

You develop Calm and Concentration and Insight by sitting still in solitude—they are literally the practice of meditation. Tantra and Ethics are the direct application of meditation. The cool, clear calm of Calm and Concentration and Insight are balanced with the juice, fire and ecstasy of Tantra.

Being still and seeing clearly

When you practise meditation for Calm and Concentration, you develop the ability to relax and balance yourself whenever you choose. You explore the states of absorption and experience the mind and body at their most peaceful, still and blissful. In Insight meditation you directly experience the fundamental nature of the mind and consciousness, then the fundamental nature of the world, and the relationship between the two.

Practising meditation largely depends on being still on your own, because to see clearly, the mind needs to be completely still and balanced. The strengths of Calm and Concentration and Insight meditation are that you develop inner calm, emotional and mental health, self-reliance and the ability to see through all the stories and beliefs we have about ourselves and life. They lead you to experience what Buddhism calls *ultimate truth*—the universal laws.

Warmth and relationship

Having experienced ultimate truth what do you do with it? You may be very calm and clear but not have any real warmth. You might have seen the truth, but that was one moment in time, and what about now?

This is where the other two streams come into play. They form the application of the skills of Calm and Concentration and Insight in our bodies, here and now. They focus on how we relate to other people and the world. Buddhism calls this *relative truth*—the laws of relationship. *Ultimately* we are all transient, ever-changing, not solid or separate, and we create our own view of reality. *Relatively* we have to eat and we depend on each other for our survival and quality of life.

Emotional freedom

Tantra and Ethics provide the means to apply the cool calm gained from Calm and Concentration and Insight to everyday life through developing tolerance and compassion for others. We are able to see where they are instead of assuming we know. We can apply the experiences of Insight to our lives so that our actions work with others rather than against them. Tantra and Ethics develop the heart, the feeling of being intimately connected with everyone and everything, so they are not learned in solitude but within all the relationships of our lives.

Tantra specialises in taking the emotions that were cooled down through Calm and Concentration and Insight and deliberately heating them up again. It's based on the understanding that nothing happens by chance—everything we are and experience arises through the conditions that support our lives, so even our most distorted and painful emotions have a reason for their existence. Although we can't change what has happened, we can change what is happening by learning how to tap the energy driving these emotions and using it skillfully.

Tantra also brings the bliss of the body and the realisations of Insight into union, so we don't drift off into blissful indulgence or dessicate in sterile intelligence. Tantra balances dry, cool clarity with moisture and warmth.

Making it your own

When you have learned the skills to develop Calm and Concentration and Insight, you can do most of it on your own. In Insight, you need a teacher to check and test the experiences that arise, but only at those times. Because Tantra is relationship—with yourself, your body, emotions and mind, and with everyone around you—a teacher helps provide a focus for this. Like all relationships it can be healthy, unhealthy or a mixture of both, so it depends on understanding where the responsibilities lie and establishing a healthy, ethical basis for its development.

This relationship does not need to become dependent, or permanent. The teacher's responsibility is to point to the clear, spacious centre of every emotion and experience, so that you experience what it's like to bring bliss and warmth together with the cool clarity of openness. Through this you come to know your inner teacher; the process becomes internalised and you can sustain it yourself.

The Lifeflow Technique

The next three books in this series are dedicated to the streams of Insight, Tantra and Ethics—together they form the whole package of the meditation tradition. Lifeflow Meditation teaches all four streams because when you take just one aspect you get a very limited idea and experience of what meditation actually is and what it can be used for. Students often attempt to develop a practice based on just one stream, which can become unbalanced and frustrating.

This is often a serious fault in teaching as well. For example, teaching only Calm and Concentration can produce the foggy, spaced-out state that is popularly associated with meditation (meditation as a drug). Teaching Insight without Calm and Concentration can lead to an idealised practice completely disassociated from life and the body, which can produce a hard, arrogant view of life (meditation as a shield).

Teaching Tantra without the other streams can, quite simply, create chaos. It's similar to doing chemistry experiments without the protection of a laboratory. And Ethics without the clarity of Insight and warmth of Tantra becomes, as nearly all ethics are, a set of commandments that may or may not have anything to do with the reality of our lives.

Calm and Concentration and Insight are for the mind; Tantra and Ethics are for the body. If you want the basic skills of meditation to train your mind and emotions, to achieve a relaxed, calm and alert state whenever you want, then learning the basics of the first two streams is all that is necessary.

The basic course, Level 1 of the Lifeflow Meditation technique, teaches these skills—focusing the mind so you can relax immediately and become calm and develop awareness in both meditation and everyday situations. However, it also includes basic steps to lay the foundation for developing the absorptions, Insight meditation and the exercises of Tantra and Ethics.

Level 2 introduces the structures, ideas and practice necessary to understand and develop the four streams. You are introduced to the levels of absorption, the steps for Insight meditation and the ideas and exercises of Tantra and Ethics.

In Level 3, the four streams form the structure of the course, which provides all the theory and exercises necessary to develop them, understand how they work and apply them. This continues in Level 4 at an advanced level.

In all, the Lifeflow Technique is a five-year program that provides training in the four streams in an Australian form, which is easy to understand and apply. It retains the depth and richness of the tradition, and anyone prepared to undertake the discipline of a regular practice can draw from this rich well of knowledge and experience.

Together the four streams form an integrated whole which is the most wonderful, enriching, wise and clear-seeing discipline I have ever met. It's not based on ideas, beliefs, theories or experiments on something or someone else. It's a way to know yourself, the human mind and your emotions through *your own direct experience*.

It has been my privilege to train thousands of people in the basics of meditation, hundreds in the more advanced practices and a group of seven teachers who are now my colleagues in the Centre. With great pleasure I have also guided many students through the levels of Insight and the experiences and realisations of Tantra.

Epilogue

At the end of a recent Level 1 course, a student asked what I had gained from meditation and I replied that it had enabled me to maintain my emotional and mental wellbeing. She wasn't satisfied with that answer! On reflection, although the answer meant a lot to me because I understood its implications, it didn't provide the whole picture.

If I had not met the meditation tradition I would have remained a professional musician and it would have been a wonderful life—doing something I loved, having power and recognition, being reasonably wealthy and protected. But I would have felt internally empty and I couldn't ignore this; I had tried everything.

Externally I would have been charming, ambitious and successful, with enough determination to make the hard decisions. Internally I would have been left with a sense of yearning I could never have satisfied.

Meditation provided the tool to tap the richness, joy, bliss and immediacy of life itself, and to feel this right through my mind and body. I've been able to explore the entire range of emotional life, from the deepest despair to the highest ecstasy, and take the fear out of emotions I didn't want to experience.

Developing calm and concentration has enabled me to be self-contained and experience the deep peace of being balanced and still. Insight meditation provided me with the discipline to achieve mental stability and clarity to the point where I could experience the ultimate nature of the human mind and how it works. It led me to an understanding of human consciousness beyond anything I could have imagined. It also brought my thinking and feeling together instead of being in conflict. Seeing clearing that everything in life is transient freed me from the pain of clinging and yearning.

Through Tantra I discovered what used to be called the *elixir of life* or *fountain of youth*. It also provided a way to discover and keep in touch with the depth of my being and the tools to live in my body and develop rich emotional resources. And, although I was given a good ethical basis in my home and community, the Ethics stream of meditation has enabled me to understand how to act skillfully, and the true meaning of love and compassion.

Through studying and teaching meditation I have met people from all walks of life and I find I can communicate with anyone and everyone on their own terms—it's a dance I thoroughly enjoy.

Meditation opens up a way of life free from the beliefs and constraints we habitually lock ourselves in. It has freed me from having to believe my own stories about myself. I discovered that my happiness lay in my own heart and hands. This is our natural heritage—the legacy that comes to us through the incredible gift of a human mind and body.

In a way, meditation was the switch that turned on the light in my mind and body—literally. My own life became luminous. I sincerely hope that if and when you decide to develop a meditation practice, you will find the illumination and joy which became part of my life.

Notes

[1] Williams, G. 2008. *Insight and Love*. Australia: Lifeflow Meditation Centre.

[2] Weill, A. 1997. *Spontaneous Healing*. USA: Time Warner, p.264.

[3] O'Connor, J. and Seymour, J. 1993. *Introducing Neuro-Linguistic Programming*. London: The Aquarian Press.

[4] Gur, R. cited in Pease, A. and Pease, B. 1998. *Why Men Don't Listen and Women Can't Read Maps*. Australia: Pease Training International, p.22.

[5] DeLosAngeles, D., Williams, G., Burston, J., Pope, K.J., Clark, C.R., Loveless, S., Lewis, T., Whitham, E., Fitzgibbon, S., Wallace, A. and Willoughby, J.O. 2007. *Electroencephalographic changes during states of Buddhist concentrative meditation*, abstract presented to 7th International Brain Research Organisation World Congress of Neuroscience, Melbourne, 12–17 July.

[6] Fox, M. 1980. Breakthrough: *Meister Eckhart's Creation Sprituality in New Translation*. New York: Doubleday, Image, pp.75-77.

[7] Chalmers, D. J. Dec. 1995. 'The Puzzle of Conscious Experience' in *Scientific America*, vol. 12, no. 1. pp.62–68.

[8] The Rolling Stones. 2002. *Rolling Stones Forty Licks*. Audio CD. Virgin/ABKCO/Decca. Disc 1.

[9] Ellis, A. 2002. *Late Night Live* interview with Phillip Adams on 25 June 2002. ABC.

[10] *Brain Story*. 2001. ABC video recording, BBC.

[11] Dijksterhuis, A., Bos, M.W., Nordgren, L. and van Baaren R.B. 2006. 'On Making the Right Choice: The Deliberation-Without-Attention Effect' in *Science* vol. 311, no. 5763, pp.1005–1007.

[12] Jung, C. G. 1960. Psychological Commentary to Evans-Wentz (ed.), *The Tibetan Book of the Dead*. London: Oxford University Press.

[13] *The Canticle of Brother Sun*. 1973. trans.Benen Fahy, O.F.M. from *St. Francis of Assisi: Writings and Early Biographies*, edited by Marion A. Habig, Franciscan Herald Press.

[14] Johnston, William (ed.). 1973. *The Cloud of Unknowing*. New York: .Doubleday, Image.

[15] Chang, G.C. 1963. *Six Yogas of Naropa and Teachings on Mahamudra*. Ithica, NY: Snow Lion Publications, pp. 38-39.

[16] Jacobs, G. D. 2003. *The Ancestral Mind*. USA: Viking Penguin,

[17] Jung, C.G. 1971. *Psychological Types*, trans. Baynes and Hull. London: Routledge and Kegan Paul.

[18] Ibid.

[19] Lutyens, M (ed), 1970. *The Penguin Krishnamurti Reader*, Penguin Books, p 171.

[20] Johnston, William op. cit.

[21] Bandler, R. and Grinder, J. 1975. *Frogs into Princes*. Real People Press.
------------1982. Reframing: *Neuro-Linguistic Programming and the Transformation of Meaning*. Real People Press.

About The Lifeflow Meditation Centre

The Lifeflow Meditation Centre is an Australian not-for-profit educational organisation founded in 1981. The Centre teaches meditation in a way that is student focused, simple and straightforward, and has taught thousands of people how to meditate. Its high quality courses and retreats have attracted local, national and international students. The Lifeflow Meditation technique is extremely practical, free from belief and jargon and easily accessible so that it can be readily integrated with everyday life. All the teachers have at least ten years of training, teach from their own experience, give personal guidance, and can answer directly in plain English any questions students may have. The introductory courses have proven very popular with people from all walks of life.

Courses

At The Lifeflow Meditation Centre's city studio, public meditation courses are run all week. There are four levels from introductory, which comprises one class per week over 7 weeks, to the advanced course. The classes are held in a spacious, well-lit room.

The Lifeflow introductory course (Level 1) provides all the experience and information needed to learn how to meditate. It covers all the different kinds of meditation so that everyone can find the type which suits them. Each class explores a different topic which explains the theory behind meditation, so you not only learn how to meditate but also what you are doing and why. The classes explain:

- what meditation actually is
- the different categories of meditation
- the deeper levels you experience
- how to develop awareness through meditation and use this in everyday life
- how to turn daily activities into short meditations
- how to improve concentration
- how to manage strong emotions
- how meditation relates to health, and
- how meditation can be used to develop your intuition.

The Level 2 course builds on the knowledge and experience gained in Level 1 and spends three terms, each of 7 weeks, exploring a particular topic and developing it in detail. Each term is a self-contained module—you can do just one to suit yourself or follow through the three modules of this level. The modules explore the topics of *The skill of mindfulness, Developing meditative concentration* and *Balancing life*. As with the Level 1 course there is plenty of time set aside for practice.

In Level 3 practice and theory are linked (as in Levels 1 and 2) so that you gain knowledge and understanding of the experiences that unfold as you build your meditation practice. Everything taught at the Lifeflow Centre is based on the direct experience of meditation, so it is accessible and immediately applicable to your life. The classes involve active discussion and practice and each term is a self-contained module. This Level spans 8 modules over two years and covers the four streams of the meditation tradition: Calm and Concentration, Insight, Tantra and Ethics.

The advanced classes of Level 4 explore in detail the highest levels of the philosophy and psychology of the meditation tradition in a practical, straightforward and simple way. This knowledge is integrated with the Western philosophical and psychological traditions as there are many aspects of both which are complementary. As always, both theory and practice are linked to the realities of everyday life. This course is intended for students who have a well-established personal meditation practice and spans 8 modules over two years, covering the four streams of the meditation tradition.

Retreats

The Centre has two retreat properties.

Tara Hills Retreat Centre, our principal retreat centre, is set amongst rolling hills, native gum trees and an abundance of bird life in the serenity and beauty of Native Valley (near Nairne in the Adelaide Hills). Purpose-built meditation buildings offer individual rooms and communal halls. Nourishment for the mind is accompanied by freshly prepared food for the body.

Tara Hills is only 40 minutes from Adelaide and regular public retreats are run there, from weekend retreats to ten-day retreats. Retreat themes include *Balancing Life, Transforming Emotions, The Joy of*

Being, Dreams—myth and reality, The Dark Night of the Soul , Health and Healing, Developing Awareness, Vitality, Wisdom, Experiencing Union, Riding the Surfboard of Life, Insight, The Deeper States of Meditation and *Music as Meditation*.

The Kurlana Sanctuary in the Riverland, near the River Murray, comprises one thousand acres of natural scrub, which has been preserved for the wild life, and retreats are run there for members of the Centre. Members can experience bush camping in the wild beauty of original mallee, the oldest living species of tree in the world and unique to Australia. On the property is an original pioneer house, which has been restored by the Centre and provides the venue for classes and meals.

The Lifeflow Meditation Centre also offers:

- Four terms of courses each year from Level 1 to Level 4
- Retreats and workshops at Tara Hills Retreat Centre
- Customised meditation training courses at our studio or at workplaces
- Corporate programs
- Courses and sessions for schools
- Personal consultations to guide your meditation practice
- Courses for meditation guides
- Teacher training programs

For further information please contact:
The Lifeflow Meditation Centre
www.lifeflow.com.au
E: info@lifeflow.com.au
P: (61) 08 8379 9001

CDs and Books

Meditation CDs

Experience Yourself, four guided meditations by Graham Williams
The Joy of Being, guided Lifeflow Meditations with music by
renowned Australian composer Ross Edwards, ABC Classics—
available through ABC Shops and book stores.

Books

The 5-Minute Meditator, Eric Harrison, Perth Meditation Centre,
Australia, 2005
Insight and Love, Graham Williams, Lifeflow Meditation Centre,
Australia, 2007

Music CDs

Reflections in Water, piano music of Debussy, Chopin and Liszt,
played by Graham Williams
My Heart keeps Watch, piano music of Olivier Messiaen, played by
Graham Williams

Books and CDs can be paid for by cheque or credit card and
ordered from:

The Lifeflow Meditation Cente

Unit 8 / 259 Glen Osmond Rd, Frewville SA 5063, Australia
Ph (61) 08 8379 9001
www.lifeflow.com.au